Fit for Life

Other books by Suzy Prudden and Jeffrey Sussman

Suzy Prudden's Family Fitness Book

Suzy Prudden's Creative Fitness for Baby and Child

Fit for Life

Suzy Prudden's Complete Program for Getting and Staying Fit for Life

Suzy Prudden and **Jeffrey Sussman**

With photographs by Jeffrey Sussman

Macmillan Publishing Co., Inc.
New York
Collier Macmillan Publishers
London

NOTE TO READERS: It is essential that you consult a physician before trying any of the remedies and exercises contained in this book, and in no case should you try any of them without the full concurrence of your physician. It is also important that you do not discontinue the treatment and diet prescribed by your doctor.

Macmillan Publishing Co., Inc.
866 Third Avenue, New York, N.Y. 10022
Collier Macmillan Canada, Ltd.

Library of Congress Cataloging in Publication Data
Prudden, Suzy.
 Fit for life.
 Includes index.
 1. Exercise. 2. Physical fitness. I. Sussman,
Jeffrey, joint author. II. Title.
GV481.P8   613.7   78-2532
ISBN 0-02-599400-X

First Printing 1978
Printed in the United States of America

To our son Robby

Contents

Fit for Life: An Introduction

Throughout childhood and adolescence most of us took our health and fitness for granted; we may have hung out in ice-cream parlors after school, eaten junk foods during Saturday matinees at local movie theatres, and exercised or engaged in sports only when we felt like it.

Much has changed, of course, since our teen-age years, and our attitudes toward fitness have undergone radical changes. We and our contemporaries constitute the most health-conscious consumers who have ever lived. As we have grown older, advancing into our twenties and thirties, we have had to increase our awareness and improve our life-style. Reading of the frequency of cardiac arrest among those not yet out of the thirties, we have been motivated by a concern to maintain our health for as long as possible. That concern extends beyond our own lives to those of our students, and to those of you who may benefit from our book.

It is important to know that from the age of twenty-four onward your body produces fewer and fewer cells; youthfulness diminishes but it can be replaced with attractive health, vigor, and strength. You may be skeptical, but we can only use ourselves as living proof. As the daughter of Bonnie Prudden, Suzy found her own special niche for rebellion when she was a teen-ager by becoming fat. Yes, fat! We mean 160 pounds of rebellion. Emerging from her teen-age years, she suddenly shed forty-five pounds and saw that her mother's attitude toward fitness was not at all obnoxious. At the age of thirty-four, she now weighs 115 pounds, is lithe, limber, and has the heart and body of a youthful athlete. Suzy exercises regularly and has formulated exercise programs that are fun to do, either alone or with others.

Jeffrey, who manages our business and writes our exercise books and articles, was a thin, athletic teen-ager. Suddenly, in his twenties, he was dismayed to find himself developing a paunch.

In addition to his fifty sit-ups, I gave him some less gruelling but more effective stomach exercises which he quickly accepted. Within three weeks, not only had his paunch disappeared, but his stomach was getting flatter and as hard as he had remembered it when he swam regularly.

We note our own experience, not out of egotism, but because what has happened to us happens to millions of others. It usually begins insidiously after the age of twenty-four. The cellular structure of the body's chemistry not only changes then, but one often slides into a sedentary routine, either involving a career or a role at home.

Women usually develop spreading thighs, thickened stomachs, and heavy buttocks; men begin with paunches which then balloon into tires. Both sexes note extra chins and dewlaps, a little extra flab on the biceps, and a general diminution of energy.

It need not and should not be that way. With only twenty to thirty minutes of exercise daily, you can trim away excess fat and become the attractive, healthy person you admire. You can even skip a day here and there, and if you do not have a block of time for fitness, then you can fit it into various parts of your day. We shall show you how to exercise while speaking on the telephone, how to inconspicuously exercise while traveling, plus any number of private exercises you can do in public places. We shall show you how to be completely fit even if you work fifteen hours a day, seven days a week. Furthermore, we shall show you how to begin a fitness program regardless of what shape you are in now and of what shape you were in as a teen-ager. We shall show you how to ease your way into a jogging routine, whether it's only once around the block or three miles every morning. Finally, we can give you an eight-minute routine, done to music, which quite literally utilizes every muscle in your body. After you have gone through this book, you will have few, if any, excuses for not being fit, and you will have added years to your life. With a minimal amount of time, you should have a lean body, a strong heart, and the necessary endurance for a successful career, marriage, and life of leisure.

Just as there is a definite correlation, during one's primary and secondary school years, between mental and physical development, so there is a similar correlation throughout one's entire life. The person who is short of breath, because short of exercise, will always have a short temper during periods of stress and tension, for one's fitness helps one through periods of stress and tension. And a short temper, like a short fuse, will hardly further a career, a marriage, or even a drive in one's car.

It is our intention to deal with your entire body, to show you how to get back into shape, and how to stay there, while controlling particular problems.

We make no promises you cannot keep with yourself. We want only to inspire you and to show you how to have a long and healthy life, one built on the concept of a strong, fit body.

1

"I Grow Old. I Grow Old"

People assume that growing old means doing less, but maturity is not a synonym for inactivity. In fact, if you maintain your health, you need never give up sports, sex, work, or hobbies. We have met many people who have enthusiastically refused to settle down for blank lives of inactivity. Yet many of them had once given up sports and exercise. They found themselves caught up in the new responsibilities of careers, households, and the raising of incredibly energetic children. One day they awoke to the realization of oncoming age. Not yet out of their twenties, and they felt like pulling the covers over their heads. Evenings of exhaustion and lethargy had become a way of non-living; television, the passive entertainer, seemed the liveliest force in their households. Cellulite and fat had hit without warning, sparing neither men nor women. These friends of ours recognized the effects of inactivity and put together plans of attack.

The most successful ones were those who began with modest fitness programs and gradually increased the duration and demands of their exercises. Before very long, many were jogging, playing tennis, or swimming at health clubs. The tempo of their lives had picked up and even the quality and rate of their professional triumphs increased, for they had enhanced their energy and stamina.

So if you are not satisfied with your figure and state of fitness, it is not too late to take charge of your life. You need only begin our exercise program, and soon you will feel a new zest for life and be pleased with your improved appearance.

Each of us is affected by two kinds of aging—primary and secondary. Primary aging is the normal loss of brain cells, the drying out of the skin, and a general wearing down of the body. Secondary aging is affected by what you do to yourself. By treating yourself with kindness and thoughtfulness, you can expect to maintain an attractive, healthy body. If you overeat and omit exercise, you can expect the secondary aging process to accelerate significantly. The negative results of secondary aging may be overweight, arteriosclerosis, and even a heart that is old when it should be young.

3

Two of the worst villains affecting secondary aging are stress and tension. They cause ulcers, damaged hearts, insomnia, constipation, and other unpleasant conditions. Many people who chain smoke gamble with such dire complications as cancer and heart attacks. Moreover, smoking so accelerates the drying out of the skin that heavy smokers often have faces as lined as corduroy pants.

Exercise can not only alleviate the effects of stress and tension, but can also reduce the pace of secondary aging. Proper diet and regular exercise maintain fitness and well-being; thin and fit people live longer than fat and sedentary people.

It is important to do both isometric and isotonic exercises. The former are primarily flexing exercises, requiring little or no movement in space. The latter require vigorous movements of muscles. Each is complementary and valuable to any exercise program. You can harden your stomach by contracting abdominals, then further improve your figure with a series of sit-ups.

The Time of Your Life

Isotonic exercises provide a sensible way to increase longevity since they strengthen the heart. To be effective, though, they must be adapted to your physical condition. If you haven't exercised for some time, we strongly recommend that you first have a complete physical checkup, including a cardiogram. Your doctor should be able to tell you how much exercise is right for you and what your incremental limits are.

In our experience with people, we have observed that for every year without exercise, it takes a full month to get into optimum shape. The longer you wait, the more difficult it becomes. Though isotonic exercises, particularly the endurance ones (jogging, walking, running, swimming, and skiing), will help develop a strong and healthy heart, they should never be overdone, especially by those who have never, or rarely, exercised. Once you've been given a medical okay to proceed with an exercise program, your endurance exercises should not be prolonged beyond ten minutes. They should be comfortably and steadily paced to improve circulation and increase the quantity of oxygen carried in the bloodstream.

With a daily routine of endurance exercises, you should be able to strengthen your heart while decreasing the at-rest beat. The beat of the heart remains the key to physical fitness. If you are not very fit, only a small amount of physical activity will cause your heartbeat to increase. The heart of the physically unfit person may beat more than a hundred times a minute at rest, while that of the fit adult will beat about seventy to eighty times a minute.

Other factors can increase your heartbeat—coffee, cigarettes, alcohol, and excess weight. If you are excessively overweight, we suggest you lose some weight before you begin an exercise program. The dual burdens of overweight and exercise may be too much for your heart. And remember:

Avoid crash diets. They can be hazardous to your health. However, if you are only mildly overweight, you may begin to exercise and diet at the same time.

You can start with walking. Long-distance walking is a better heart exercise than many sports. Jogging is one of the best exercises; it strengthens the heart, enlarges the lungs, and improves the circulation. And since jogging has become such a popular activity, we have devoted a separate chapter on how to undertake a jogging program and carry it out successfully.

No matter what exercise program you undertake, be sure not to strain the limits of your body. Learn to listen to your heart and muscles. When your heart begins to pound, slow down and rest. If a muscle begins to ache, stop exercising and relax. There are four basic factors which determine how much exercise anyone should undertake: weight, muscle development, heartbeat, and blood pressure. The quality, rather than the quantity, of exercise is what's important. The quantity should always be increased steadily and thoughtfully, but never impulsively.

Quite obviously, we are strong advocates of exercise, especially those exercises which improve the heart. However, not all the exercise in the world can cure or even prevent certain kinds of heart disease. For example, diseases which are caused by diets high in cholesterol are hardly affected by exercise. In fact, improper exercising can be quite harmful to a person with arteries diseased by the presence of excessive cholesterol. Therefore, we encourage you to check your diet carefully with your doctor.

Zing Go the Heart Strings

Heart specialists generally agree that the long-term effect of stress and tension is to alter negatively the optimum functioning of the heart muscle. During periods of intense stress and tension, it is not unusual to experience an increased or irregular heartbeat. Not only is the heart affected, but the entire secondary aging process is accelerated.

You need not quietly endure such ravages to your health. If you exercise, you will have a strong and reliable heart, one more capable of dealing with stress and tension than a weak, tired heart. Because stress and tension influence our lives so strongly, we have devoted a separate chapter to them.

Heart attacks have become too common in our society. So much so that, at a recent meeting of the President's Council on Physical Fitness and Sports, a lecture and film were devoted to the problem. The meeting's report emphasized the importance of a daily regimen of healthful exercise, and the council has issued the following statement: "There is strong authoritative support for the concept that regular exercise can prevent degenerative diseases and slow down the physical deterioration that accompanies aging."

The exercises which we have described in this book are the result of years of teaching others to be fit. We have made numerous adaptations, and, in some instances, we have developed completely new ones. We believe that our exercises will prove to be of inestimable value to all those who want to get into shape and stay there.

Test Your Heartbeat

To test your heartbeat, place the first two fingers of your right hand on your carotid artery, which is located on the right side of your throat. Now count the number of pulsations for fifteen seconds and multiply the number by four. The total is your heartbeat per minute. A healthy heart should beat about seventy-five beats per minute for men and about eighty beats per minute for women. Your heartbeat should be faster after exercise but return to normal within a short period of time after resting. If your heartbeat is significantly faster than the above, then you're potentially in trouble and need the advice of your doctor. You'll have to slow down your exercise rate and check your diet carefully. One cup of coffee can increase your heartbeat (in some cases) by ten beats per minute. Remember, it is imperative to see your doctor for a cardiogram before commencing any exercise program, regardless of how healthy you think you are.

HEARTBEAT TEST

Daily Day & date started	Time	AM at rest	Standing	After normal activity	After exercise	10 min. after exercise	PM at rest

Periodically Date started							
After 4 wks.							
After 3 mos.							
After 6 mos.							
After 1 yr.							

2

Getting Fit for Fitness

No one's body should be flung into an exercise program without first realizing its capabilities. Once you've gotten your doctor's authorization to begin exercising, you should next examine what it is you want from an exercise program. The most reliable judge is your mirror, which can tell you the truth about yourself. Never forget, the human body is malleable and can be sculptured by proper exercise.

Next, you should take your measurements (as listed at the back of this chapter) and decide what you want them to be. Don't shoot for the moon; unrealistic goals will simply end in frustration. Begin your program by simply walking and doing basic warm-up exercises (also to be found at the conclusion of this chapter, along with a test for minimum strength and flexibility).

If you prefer jogging instead of walking, remember not to do too much. If your muscles tense with pain or your heart beats too fast, then stop.

You need not jog more than a quarter of a mile to begin with, and, if that is too tiring, you can walk fifty steps, jog fifty steps. Continue the alternation until you feel sufficiently strong to jog without walking fifty steps. However, you should never jog, then run, for the strain on your heart may be too great.

If done with care, jogging and walking are superb endurance exercises which improve circulation, strengthen the heart, and give extra boosts of oxygen to the brain. Jogging may actually raise your I.Q.

More to the point of your life, though, you will experience an overall sense of health and vigor; your entire demeanor will take on a new aspect of youthfulness. All you need do is exercise.

Time and Time Again

All exercises, regardless of the kinds, should be done for ten to thirty minutes *daily* and for the same amount of time each day. The exercises should be sufficiently rigorous to increase your strength, coordination, flexibility, and endurance.

Increase your exercises incrementally. No matter how enthusiastic you may feel one day, do not increase your amount of exercise too quickly. And remember, one kind of exercise is no substitute for another. Push-ups cannot replace the effects of sit-ups, and neither sit-ups nor push-ups, by themselves, are sufficient to keep your entire body in shape.

Exercise is a process which, if done on a regular basis, can improve the quality of your life.

Mountains of Muscles

Before we go on into other areas, we believe you should have more detailed knowledge of muscles. You will be able to exert greater control over your own development by knowing what it is you are exercising.

The more than 300 muscles in the human body comprise about half of each person's weight. Muscles not only move every part of the body (from eyeballs to intestines to legs), but they keep stomachs flat and prevent lower back pain. Muscles are divided into two groups, voluntary and involuntary.

The voluntary muscles are the ones you can exercise, either isometrically or isotonically, and they are stimulated by your nervous system. Every time you take a step or move a finger, your brain sends out the appropriate signal. When held in a commonly relaxed state, the voluntary muscles are only partly contracted; when signaled by the brain, they contract suddenly, moving limbs in a flash. In order for your voluntary muscles to work well, they should be well-toned, flexible, and strong.

Involuntary muscles are much smoother than voluntary ones. This group of muscles is in the intestines and arterial walls, enabling one to eat, breathe, and maintain vital bodily functions. The heart, of course, is one of the most important involuntary muscles. It can be toned and strengthened by endurance exercises. With the help of a nutritious diet low in cholesterol and fats, the coronary arteries can be kept free from arteriosclerosis.

If you could peel away your envelope of skin, you could see a complicated network of voluntary muscles. In the well-toned, well-exercised body, their design is as perfect as their utility and seems the perfect work of a great sculptor.

A Lineup of Volunteers

Below, we briefly list the most important voluntary muscles which must be utilized in any successful exercise program.

Sternomastoid: These are found on both sides of the neck and are essential not only for poise and balance, but because they enable you to move your neck with grace and flexibility. They are especially noticeable in soccer players who must often use their heads—and not just for thinking.

Deltoids: These are the muscles which cover the tops of the shoulders. Well-toned deltoids result in smooth, attractive shoulders.

Trapezius. Some people wish they did not have this muscle, for it is often an area known for its sharp pain. It is triangular in shape and spreads across

8

the back from shoulders to neck. You need not experience contractions in the
trapezius if you know how to relax that muscle.

Biceps. These are the muscles at the fronts of the upper arms which weight lifters seem to love irrationally. The biceps should be well developed, for they are essential in controlling the arms and fingers.

Triceps. These are not three biceps; they are important muscles located on the backs of the upper arms. When they are well-toned, they give the arms a streamlined look.

Pectorals. These may be the second most beloved muscles of weight lifters; however, they are even more important to women, for pectorals are the chest muscles beneath a woman's breasts. If a woman wants larger breasts, she need only develop her pectorals for both size and support. In men, well-toned pectorals give an appearance of firmness and strength.

Serratus anterior. Not the name of a Roman gladiator or a Latin maxim. Rather, they are the muscles on either side of the upper rib cage that provide strength for essential pushing movements performed by the arms.

Abdominals. These muscles are particularly well-developed by swimmers. The abdominals are not a pair of muscles, but an entire group, including the obliques and transversalis. When properly developed, they form three strong layers, extending from the diaphragm to the pelvis, where they act as a natural girdle.

Rectus abdominus. Not the name of a Latin contortionist, but those muscles which are part of the abdominal structure. They are located down the middle of the stomach and continue to the pubic bone. They are vital to the bending motions of the body's trunk.

Psoas. This refers to either of two muscles located on both sides of the loin. Extending from the sides of the spinal column, they terminate at the femur in the thigh. The psoas is essential to the process of drawing up the thighs as well as to pelvic movement.

All exercises which include the last three muscles will increase flexibility and endurance during sexual intercourse. (We shall devote an entire chapter to sexercises.)

Gluteal muscles. These comprise the entire buttock area of the body. When not properly toned, they contribute to a fat, lumpy figure. The most commonly known of the gluteals is the largest, the gluteus maximus, located nearest to the surface of the skin.

The Hamstrings. Most people who sit at a desk all day can be made suddenly aware of their hamstrings by suddenly standing up and trying to touch their toes. A groan of pain is the usual reaction. The hamstrings are located in the backs of the thighs, and they often contract from lack of use. (At the end of this chapter are limbering and warm-up exercises which will stretch and loosen your hamstrings.)

Quadriceps femoris. These muscles, located in the front of the thighs, are extremely important to those who jog, run, or walk for endurance. Soccer players, track athletes, gymnasts, and dancers all have very well-developed quadriceps.

Calves. The calf muscle is one of the most obviously pronounced muscles of the human anatomy, and it often experiences pain during periods of stress and exhaustion. People with poor circulation often experience the sensation of pins-and-needles in their calves. The effects on the calves of stress, exhaustion, and poor circulation can be minimized by exercise, and jogging is one of the best.

These muscles are not all the muscles in the human body, but, aside from the heart, they are the ones which we are most concerned with exercising. Should it be necessary, for a particular sport, to develop additional muscles, we will discuss it at the appropriate time. While exercising the most obvious groups of muscles, you will also be exercising lesser groups, for no single muscle operates independently. The result should be muscles as long, lean, and elegant as a cheetah's. Such muscles are far more useful than the bulky muscles on a weight lifter's body.

Arriving Where We Started

On the following page, you will find the Kraus-Weber Test for Minimum Strength and Flexibility. You should take it without worrying, for it is a simple test. It will provide you with an opportunity to test the basic strength and flexibility of the muscles we have discussed above. If you pass the test, you can begin a regular, ten-minute-daily exercise program, but if you discover weaknesses, you should start with special exercises to strengthen particular parts of your body.

We have also provided a chart in which you can write down your measurements. It is *your* chart, and no one else need see it. It is to chart your progress to your own goals, and these goals should be realistically set, based on what you are not only capable of accomplishing, but also on what you are ultimately comfortable with. As you proceed with your exercise program, you will be able to judge your progress, and there is nothing more satisfying than having proof of your successful commitment to self-improvement.

Rules of the Game

After you have checked your problem areas and have decided where you want to make specific improvements, pick out the exercises most suitable to your needs. Read each exercise through before you attempt it. Always begin with five minutes of warm-up exercises and then add twenty minutes of regular exercises. The last five minutes are a period for slowing down, and they should be devoted to stretchercises and relaxercises to avoid weakness or stiffness.

Happy Times

The exercise program which we have carefully put together should not be tedious. It should and will be fun, a time which will give you pleasure. However, before you begin, you can insure your enjoyment and effectiveness by
following these rules.

First, wear something comfortable, be careful not to choose garments which are either too tight or too constricting.

Second, put on some of your favorite music; use a tempo that gives you bounce, but one that you can keep up with without experiencing either discomfort or fatigue.

Third, always warm up your muscles. After a few minutes of warm-up exercises your body is primed to function to capacity and is far less susceptible to injury.

Fourth, never exercise when you're not in the mood for it; if you do, you will resent it as much as you may have resented homework. Find a time during the day when you can really enjoy and benefit from your exercise program.

Kraus-Weber Test

	Date & time of day	HF	A&HF	A-HF	UB	LB	Flex.
Beginning							
After 4 wks.							
After 3 mos.							
After 6 mos.							
After 9 mos.							
After 1 yr.							

WEAK HIP FLEXORS (HF)

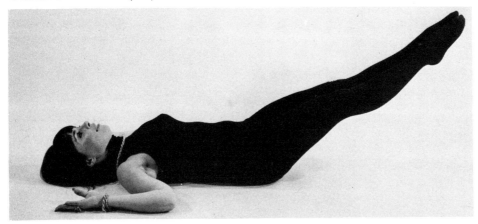

Lie supine, placing your hands next to your neck. Keeping your legs straight, raise them 10 inches off the floor and hold them in that position for 11

(cont'd)

10 seconds. If you can do this, mark the chart in the appropriate box with a check mark. If you cannot hold your legs up for the entire 10 seconds, then write down the number of seconds you were able to manage. If you are unable to lift your legs off the floor at all, then mark down a 0.

WEAK HIP FLEXORS AND ABOMINALS (A AND HF)   *spelling*

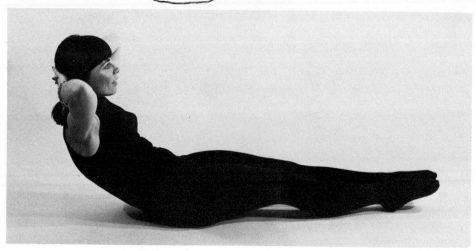

Lie supine with legs straight out and feet secure under a couch or a chair and hands clasped behind your neck. Now sit up slowly. If you can do this, mark the appropriate box with a check. If you are unable to sit up, then mark the box with a 0.

WEAK ABDOMINALS (A-HF)

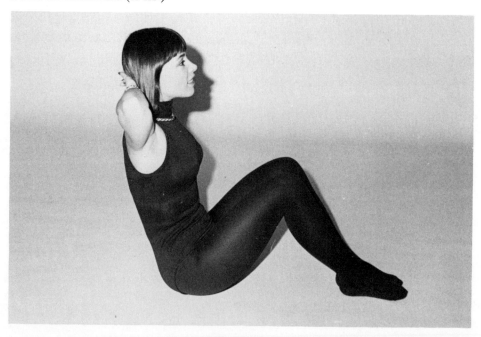

Lie supine with legs bent at the knees, feet secure under a couch or a chair, and hands clasped behind your neck. Now gently sit up. If you can do

12

this, then mark the appropriate box with a check. If you are unable to sit up, then mark the box with a 0.

WEAK UPPER BACK (UB)

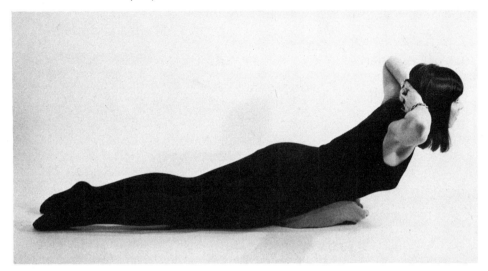

Lie prone with a pillow placed under your pelvic area and your feet held down securely (under a couch or a chair). Place your hands behind your neck and lift your torso off the floor. Hold this position for 10 seconds. If you pass, then mark a check in the appropriate box. If you cannot hold your torso up for the entire 10 seconds, then write down the number of seconds you were able to manage. If you are unable to lift your torso off the floor, then mark down a 0.

WEAK LOWER BACK (LB)

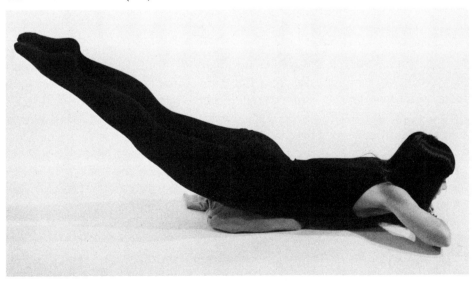

Lie prone with a pillow placed under your pelvic area and have someone gently press against your upper back so that your chest remains against the   13
(cont'd)

floor. With torso secure, and legs absolutely straight, lift those straight legs off the floor and hold the position for 10 seconds. If you pass, then mark a check in the appropriate box. If you cannot hold your legs in the air for the entire 10 seconds, then write down the number of seconds you were able to manage. If you are unable to lift your legs into the air, then mark down a 0.

LACK OF FLEXIBILITY
CAUSED BY TENSION AND
STIFFNESS (FLEX)

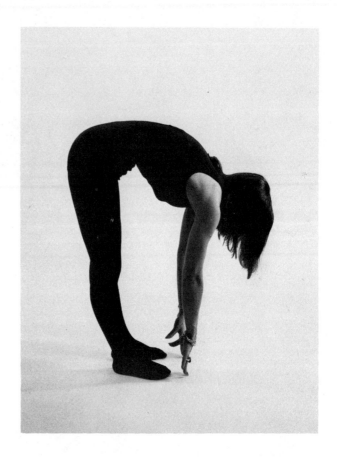

Stand with your feet together and your legs absolutely straight. Now slowly bend forward lowering your fingertips to the floor. See how close your fingers can come to the floor without bending your knees. If you can touch the floor, then mark a T in the appropriate box. If you can go further than touching with just your fingertips (e.g., touching the floor with the backs of your fists or your palms), then mark a T-plus in the box. If you cannot touch the floor, then use a ruler and see how far away from the floor your fingers are. Mark the box with a minus preceding the number of inches between your fingertips and the floor (e.g., if you can only reach to within 2 feet of the floor, mark -24).

Important: Don't bounce your way down. That's cheating, and it won't help you to accurately test yourself. And don't use the excuse that your legs are too long or that your arms are too short. Actually, if you can't touch the floor, then the muscles in the backs of your legs are too tight and too tense and need to be made more flexible.

Exercises to Improve Results of Performance on the K-W Minimum Fitness Test

WEAK HIP FLEXORS (HF)

1. Back flat—leg-lower

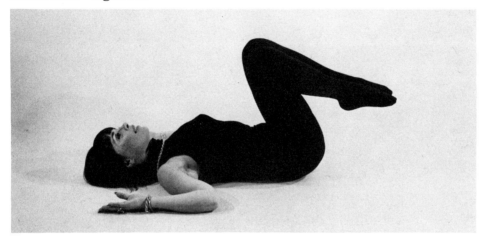

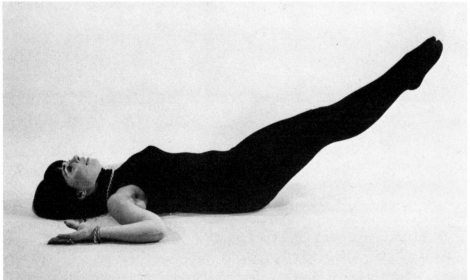

This exercise is essential for lower-back strength. If you feel pain in your lower back, then check to make sure you are doing the exercise correctly. Lie supine. Bring your knees up over your chest and then straighten your legs so that they form a 90-degree angle with your torso and the floor. Keeping the small of your back pressed firmly against the floor, slowly lower your legs. Be very careful to lower them *only* as far as you can *without* your back rising off the floor; if you feel your back rising, you have lowered your legs too far. When you reach that point, hold the position for 4 seconds, then release it by bending your knees over your chest. Rest and repeat 4 times. *Never* lower your legs all the way down to the floor, that will cause back strain. Be sure you go only as far as you can while keeping your back *flat*.

15

2. Roll-downs

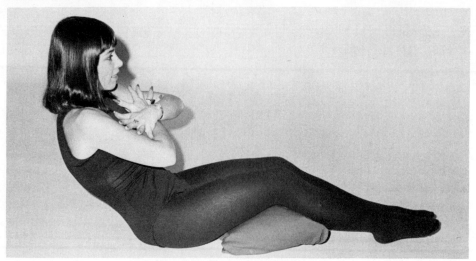

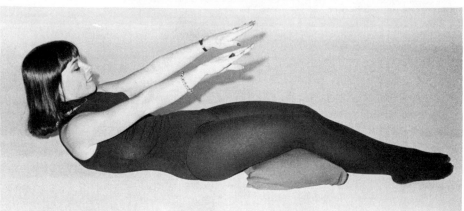

Place a pillow under your knees and insert the fronts of your feet under a couch or dresser; cross your arms on your chest. Begin in a sitting position, then slowly roll down to a supine position. Carefully try to sit up, thrusting your arms above your head and swinging them forward. Your arms will help to create momentum, pulling your body up into a sitting position. If this is too difficult, use your hands for support. Roll down again. Do 8 roll-downs, counting out 4 seconds as you lower your body. After the first week, try the sit-up again. Once you can do it easily, add 8 sit-ups to your 8 roll-downs. Once the roll-downs and sit-ups have become easy, you're ready for the next step. Place your hands behind your neck and roll down; keep your hands clasped behind your neck and sit up. Start with 1 or 2 and work up to 8 times daily, adding a few each week.

WEAK ABDOMINALS (A-HF)

3. Roll-downs with knees bent

Do the above exercise in the same progression, only bending your knees so that your legs form a triangle with the floor.

4. Prone—arm-lifts

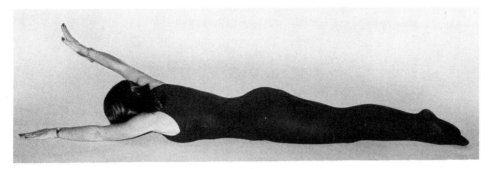

Lie prone with your chin on the floor and your arms stretched out straight in front of you. Lift your right arm into the air as high as you can, keeping it next to your ear. Your chin should remain on the floor. Lower your right arm, then lift the left arm in the same manner. Repeat 16 times.

5. Corner push-ups

Stand with your feet together facing a corner of a room at a distance of about 2 to 3 feet. Place your palms against each wall of the corner, keeping your arms at shoulder height. With your body straight, lean forward, bringing your face and chest as close to the corner as possible, then push off, back to an erect position. Repeat 8 times, making sure your elbows remain at shoulder height at all times.

6. Prone—leg-lifts

Lie prone, resting your chin on folded arms. Keeping your hipbones on the floor, raise your right leg without bending the knee. Hold the leg in the air for 2 seconds, then lower it. Raise your left leg in the same manner. Repeat 16 times.

7. Donkey-kick—knee-to-nose

Get on your hands and knees, keeping arms straight. Bring your right knee up under your body. Try to touch your nose by bringing your face down

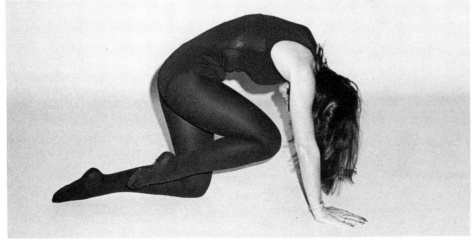

17

(cont'd)

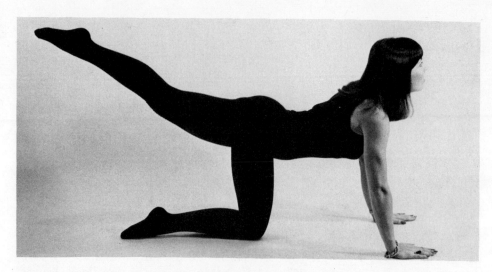

to meet your knee. Kick your leg out behind you, raising it as high as you can while lifting your head. Repeat 6 times, then repeat exercise with left leg.

LACK OF FLEXIBILITY (FLEX)

8. Standing—forward bounce

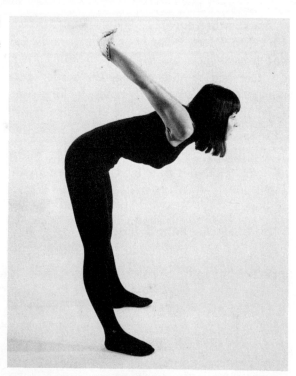

Stand with feet apart, legs straight, and hands clasped behind you. Bounce forward, bending at the hips, as low as you comfortably can without bending your knees. Keeping your arms straight, bring your hands up behind you as you bounce forward. Bounce 8 times forward, then 8 times over the right leg, 8 times forward, 8 times over the left leg, and, finally, 8 times forward again. Be sure to keep your legs straight.

9. Sitting—forward bounce, legs straight, feet together

Sit on the floor with your legs straight out in front of you and your feet together. Hold your calves, then pull your torso forward and release it back-ward. You should feel a stretching in the backs of your legs. Repeat the exercise 16 times with your toes pointed. Then flex your feet so that your toes point toward the ceiling and bounce forward and back 16 times.

Optimum Fitness Test

Caution: This test is designed only to measure what you can accomplish with ease and comfort from the time you begin your fitness program until you reach your realistic goals. When you first take the test, don't attempt more than the eight-month goals. As for jogging, stick to a quarter of a mile or less, unless you've been in a jogging program already. The day after you take the test, you will probably feel quite stiff, so begin the exercise program slowly as if you hadn't taken it at all. This way you will build up strength, coordination, and flexibility. When you take the test again in four weeks, you will see and feel significant improvements. In addition, you will not be as stiff during the following days as you had previously been.

SIT-UPS (A)

In the space allotted on the chart, mark the number of sit-ups you can do with your knees bent and hands clasped behind your neck. Have someone hold your feet down or place them under a secure object. If you twist your body, leading with one side or the other, then make a note of which side you lead with and add a few extra sit-ups, this time leading with the other side.

ONE-LEGGED KNEE-BEND (OLKB)

In the space allotted on the chart, mark approximately how low you can go and how many knee-bends you can do while standing on one leg. First test your right leg, then your left leg.

PUSH-UPS (P)

In the space allotted on the chart, mark how many push-ups you can do; be sure your body is absolutely straight.

CHIN-UPS (C)

In the space allotted on the chart, mark how many chin-ups you can do, both overhand and underhand. Do the overhand first, then do a different test exercise, returning to the underhand grip after your arms have been suffi-ciently rested.

UPPER BACK (UB)

In the space allotted on the chart, mark the number of times you can do these chest lifts. Place a pillow on top of a low box—about 6 to 8 inches high—and lie prone with your pelvic area over the pillow. The box should be placed beneath you as in the Kraus-Weber test, and your chest and knees should be resting on the floor. Someone with sufficient strength should hold

19

(cont'd)

OPTIMUM FITNESS TEST

This chart is to be used with the Optimum Fitness Test. Read through the test and then use the chart to mark your present state of fitness as well as progress.

	Date	S	OLKB		P	C	UB	LB	SF	BJ	SR	HF	W	J
			R	L										
Beg.														
4 wks.														
3 mos.														
6 mos.														
9 mos.														
1 yr.														
1½ yrs.														

BODY REACTIONS AFTER TAKING OFT

	Date	PR* before	PR* after	PR* 10 min. after	Note how does body feel?	1st day following Stiffness? Where?	2nd day following Stiffness? Where?
Beg.							
4 wks.							
3 mos.							
6 mos.							
9 mos.							
1 yr.							

* Mark in heartbeat per minute

your buttocks and legs in place. Clasp your hands behind your neck and raise and lower your torso, holding it in the raised position for 5 seconds before lowering it each time.

LOWER BACK (LB)

In the space allotted on the chart, mark the number of times you can do the following: Lie prone placing the box you used for the chest lifts under your pelvic area with your chest and knees resting on the floor. Put your forehead on your folded arms and be sure someone holds your torso down. Now straighten your legs and raise and lower them together. Hold your straight legs in the air for 5 seconds, then lower them.

SHOULDER FLEXIBILITY (SF)

In the space allotted on the chart, mark the approximate distance your arms can go back while doing the following. Hold a 3-foot dowel by each end in front of you. Raise the dowel up and continue moving it up over your head while keeping your arms straight. Stretch your arms as far back as possible without forcing them beyond a point of comfort. Eventually you should be able to do a full shoulder rotation.

BROAD JUMP (BJ)

In the space allotted on the chart, mark the number of feet you can jump starting in a stationary position and landing with your feet next to one another.

SHUTTLE RUN (SR) (for speed and coordination)

In the space allotted on the chart, mark the number of seconds it takes you to do the following exercise. Place 2-hand–sized objects 30 feet from you. Run back and forth from the starting line to the objects, picking up one object per trip and putting it on the starting line. Don't throw the objects at the starting line.

HAMSTRING FLEXIBILITY (HF)

In the space allotted on the chart, mark the number of inches past the "floor touch" you can reach without bending your knees. Stand on a box and use a ruler to measure how far down your fingers can reach past the top of the box.

WALKING (W)

How far do you walk each day? Mark down the approximate number of blocks you feel comfortable with before tiring.

JOGGING (J)

Go easy the first day and don't jog more than a quarter of a mile even if you feel you can do more. Do not run. Set a slow steady pace, slightly faster than a walk but slower than a trot. If you experience any difficulty after jogging only 50 or even 20 steps, *stop* and mark it down. This test is meant only to give you an idea of your fitness. You are competing against no one. You have plenty of time to work up to a mile or two. Don't try too much too soon.

Optimum fitness test goals after eight months

If you can do more comfortably, go ahead, but don't push yourself.

Sit-ups (A): 30 in 1 minute (knees must be bent)
One-legged knee-bend (OLKB): 6 each leg, all the way down
Push-ups (P): 30 to 50
Chin-ups (C): 20 to 30 (underhand and overhand, but no more than 40 to 100)
Upper back (UB): 25 lifts
Lower back (LB): 25 lifts
Shoulder flexibility (SF): full shoulder rotation, arms straight in front of you to straight in back, resting dowel on buttocks
Broad jump (BJ): 6 to 8 feet
Shuttle run (SR): 15 to 20 seconds
Hamstring flexibility (HF): plus 5 or 6 inches
Walking (W): unlimited
Jogging (J): 3 miles

If you intend to start with the eight-month goal in the first few weeks of your fitness program, you're risking physical trouble. If you're patient, you'll reach your goals slowly. If it takes you longer than eight months, don't worry. Your aim is a healthy body and in the end you'll achieve it.

The students at Suzy Prudden Studios Ltd. were surprised when we reported that we started our jogging program with only a quarter of a mile per day. We were up to and comfortable with a half mile after three weeks, but now we can do three miles easily, only eight months after we started. If we miss more than five days, we go back to a shorter distance and work up to three miles without endangering our health.

Measurement Chart

Measure yourself only once a month and be sure you remeasure the same areas.

To measure your arms, place a tape measure around the heaviest part of your upper arm; then measure the middle of your forearm. To measure your midriff, place the tape around your rib cage just below your breasts. Upper hips are two inches below your waist, middle hips are where your hipbones are. To measure the upper thigh, find the largest area; to measure the lower thigh, place the tape around your leg four inches above the knee. Your calves should be measured smack in the middle without contracting the muscle.

MEASUREMENT CHART

	1st day Date	4 wks. Date	8 wks. Date	3 mos. Date	4 mos. Date	5 mos. Date	6 mos. Date	7 mos. Date	8 mos. Date
Neck									
Upper right arm									
Lower right arm									
Upper left arm									
Lower left arm									
Chest									
Midriff									
Waist									
Upper hips									
Middle hips									
Lower hips									
Upper right thigh									
Lower right thigh									
Upper left thigh									
Lower left thigh									
Right knee									
Left knee									
Right calf									
Left calf									
Right ankle									
Left ankle									

Measure yourself once a month.

Once Over Lightly Figure Analysis and Posture Problem Chart

Having taken the K-W Test, your measurements, weighed yourself, and checked your heartbeat, take a good, long look at yourself, without any clothes on, in the mirror. Analyze your body's faults. Be honest or you'll do yourself an injustice. Remember, you are the one who has to face yourself each day.

Figure	*Posture* (note your problem)
OK	Upper back
Too thin	Lower back
Too heavy	Walk
Heavy all over	toe in
Heavy upper body	toe out
Heavy lower body	flat foot
Tension upper body	turned-in ankle
Tension lower body	Pain
Tension stomach	where_____
Cellulite	when_____

Exercises for particular problems. Consult chapter

a. Stomach	h. Upper back
b. Hips	i. Lower back
c. Thighs	j. Neck
d. Buttocks	k. Upper arms
e. Bustline	l. Knees
f. Waist	m. Feet
g. Midriff	n. Walk

Notes _____

_____

_____

_____

Having circled your problem areas, check the exercises for specific problems and incorporate them into your daily routine.

Exercise List

Having checked your problem areas, do the exercises listed below for each problem area. The numbers only identify the exercise. They do not indicate the number of times you should do the exercise.

a. *Stomach*
   22. Bent-knee sit-ups; 23. Bicycle; 24. On elbows—knees to chest, straighten, and circle; 187. Round back and straighten.

b. *Hips*
   50. Sitting; L position—leg-lifts; 51. Sitting; L position—leg-lift and stretch; 53. Hip-lift; 57. On knees—figure 8.

c. *Thighs*
   34. On elbow—leg lift; 35. One side—under leg-lift; 49. Infinity leg-swing; 189. On elbow—leg-bend to side, straighten leg up and then lower.

d. *Buttocks*
   6. Prone—leg-lifts; 7. Donkey-kick—knee-to-nose; 52. On hands and knees—leg-stretch; 56. Prone—leg-lift, feet apart.

e. *Bustline*
   18. The back of my hand; 19. Airplane stretch; 20. Push and pull; 21. Paint the wall.

f. *Waist*
   89. Arm swing; 135. Washing machine; 136. The touch-toe twist; 102. Overhead arm-bounce.

g. *Midriff*
   60. Elbow snap; 58. Holding hands—side-to-side bounce; 135. Washing machine; 100. Sitting, L position—side and forward bounce.

h. *Upper back*
   4. Prone—arm-lifts; 12. The swim; 16. Let-downs; 19. Airplane stretch.

i. *Lower back*
   1. Back flat—leg-lower; 6. Prone—leg-lifts; 27. Back—arch and flatten; 61. The metronome.

j. *Neck*
   10. Head roll; 78. Head twist; 79. Head back—open and close mouth; 77. Head metronome.

k. *Upper arms*
   11. Shoulder twist; 15. On knees—push-ups; 73. Shoulder rotate; 86. Shoulder circle.

l. *Knees*
   31. Half knee-bend, heel down; 32. Side-to-side knee-bend; 44. Snowplow knee-bend; 95. Deep, deep knee-bend, cross-over.

m. *Feet*
   37. Toe flex and curl; 39. Curl feet and flatten; 40. Toe stretch and release; 42 Sitting—foot flex and point.

n. *Walk*

    toe in: 208. Walk like a duck;

    toe out: 207. Walk pigeon-toed;

    flat foot: 37. Toe flex and curl, and 39. Curl feet and flatten;

    turned-in ankles: 209. Walk on the outside, and 39. Curl feet and flatten.

Once over lightly—head to toe exercises for major muscles and muscle areas:

DELTOIDS

10. Head roll

With arms at your sides, stand with your feet apart. Let your head fall forward gently without bending the upper part of your torso. Pass your right ear over your right shoulder, then let your head fall back. Move your left ear over your left shoulder, and return to the original position. Reverse the movement, going in a counterclockwise direction. Do the head roll 5 times to the right, then 5 times to the left.

11. Shoulder twist

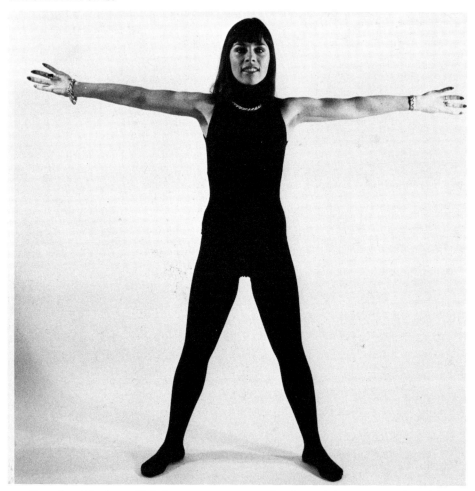

Stand with feet slightly apart, arms raised straight out to the sides at shoulder height. Stretching your arms outward, turn your palms up. Slowly

27

(cont'd)

turn your palms forward, then down, and then up behind, allowing your shoulders to rotate forward. Hold this position for 4 seconds and return to forward palms-up position for 4 seconds. Repeat 8 times.

TRAPEZIUS

12. The swim

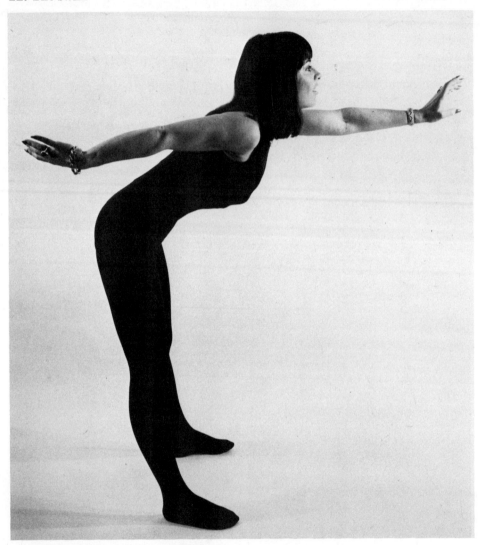

This exercise is quite simple, requiring you to move your arms as if swimming the crawl. Stand with your feet apart and bend forward from your hips. Move your arms in a swimming motion, careful to make complete circular movements. Each arm should circle 16 times.

4. Prone—arms-lifts

Lie prone with your chin on the floor and your arms stretched out straight in front of you. Lift your right arm into the air as high as you can, keeping it next to your ear and keeping your chin on the floor. Lower your right arm 28 and lift the left arm in the same manner. Repeat 16 times.

13A. Shoulders back and forth

Standing with feet together and arms at sides, push your shoulders forward, rounding them and your back. Then reverse the movement, pushing your shoulders back as far as possible. Do 16 times.

13B. The shrug

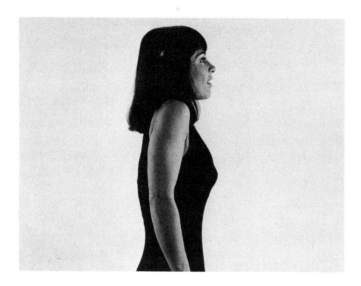

Try to raise your shoulders to your ears. Then lower your shoulders and lift your head, stretching your neck. Do 16 times.

BICEPS

14. Crab lift

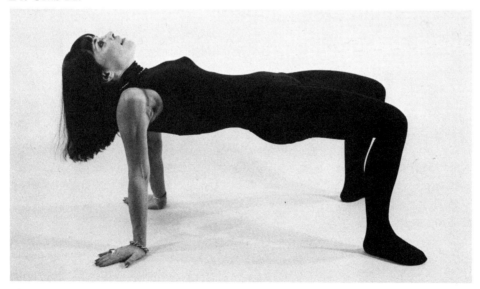

Sit on the floor with your legs apart and knees bent. Lean back and place your hands behind you, out to either side with fingertips pointing out. Lift your body off the floor, making stomach, thighs, and chest very nearly level. Your body should form a square. Arms and calves are the sides with the floor   29

(cont'd)

as the base of the square. Hold this position for 4 seconds, then relax, returning to the original position. Do 6 times.

15. On knees—push-ups

Get down on your hands and knees, but turn your hands in with fingertips facing each other. Bending your arms at the elbows, lower your body until your chin touches the floor. Now reverse the movement, raising yourself to your original position. Go up and down 16 times.

16. Let-downs

Get into the beginning push-up position, the body straight out and supported on straight arms and toes. Slowly bend your arms and lower your body to the floor, keeping your body straight and counting to 6. When you reach the floor, relax for a few seconds, then return to your starting position, but not with a push-up. Repeat the let-down 4 to 6 times, then relax.

17. Chin-ups—chin let-downs

With your hands, take hold of a bar that is directly over your head and high enough so that your arms are straight. Don't jump up. Instead, with palms forward, pull your body up until your chin is just above the bar. Slowly lower your body. Repeat 3 times and reverse your hand grip so that your palms are facing backward. Repeat the pulling motion until your chin is just above the bar; then lower your body slowly. Repeat 3 times. If this exercise proves impossible, don't despair.

Do the chin let-downs. Stand on a chair with your hands—palms forward —gripping the bar and your chin placed just above it. Your arms should be bent. Lift your feet off the chair and slowly lower your body while you count to 6 until your arms are stretched out straight. Climb back onto the chair and repeat the let-down 3 times. Change grips so that your palms are facing backward and repeat the let-down 3 more times. If you do this daily, you will soon be able to do one and then more than one chin-up.

PECTORALS

18. The back of my hand

This exercise can be done with feet either together or apart. Keep your left arm at your side and raise your right arm, bending it at the elbow. Place the back of your right hand against your right cheek. Now swing your arm, throwing your hand backwards and away from your face until your arm is as straight as a backstroker's. Do the same exercise with your left hand and arm, leaving your right at your side. Repeat 8 times with each arm.

19. Airplane stretch

Standing with feet apart, bring your arms up to shoulder height. Bend them at the elbows until your fingers touch in front of you. Quickly, but carefully, bring your elbows back as far as you can, then return them to the starting position with hands in front of you. Straighten arms out to the sides, making sure they remain at shoulder height, and turn palms upward. Return

to original position and repeat 12 times.

20. Push and pull (isometric)

Keep your elbows raised to chest height. Push your hands against each other as hard as you can and hold the position for 3 seconds. Then for another 3 seconds, try to pull your hands apart but don't let go. Repeat 8 times.

SERRATUS ANTERIOR

21. Paint the wall

Get down on your hands and knees. Imagine a can of paint on your right side and a paintbrush and a wall to paint on your left side; with your left hand reach under your right side and then swing your left hand back out toward the right, lifting it as high as you can. Do 4 times, then change arms.

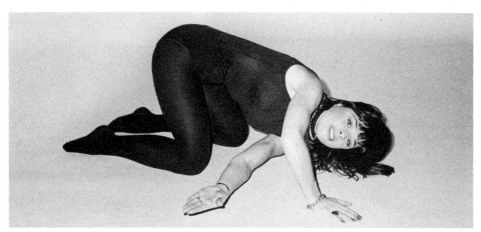

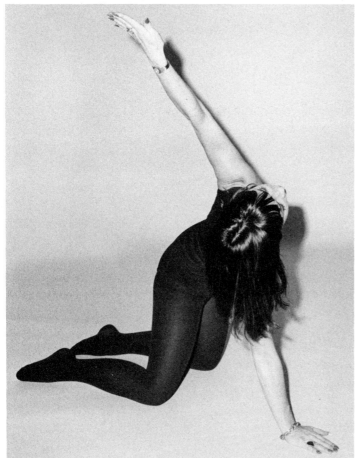

31

5. Corner push-ups

Stand with your feet together facing a corner of a room at a distance of about 2 to 3 feet. Place your palms against each wall of the corner, keeping your arms at shoulder height. Keeping your body straight, lean forward, bringing your face and chest as close to the corner as possible, then push off, back to an erect position. Repeat 8 times, making sure your elbows remain at shoulder height at all times.

ABDOMINALS

22. Bent-knee sit-ups

Sit on the floor with knees bent, placing feet under a couch, dresser, or sturdy piece of furniture. Clasp your hands behind your neck. From sitting position, lie down slowly. When your back is flat on the floor, sit up, keeping your hands clasped behind your neck. Be sure to come up with a rounded back and straighten it when you have reached the final sitting position. Begin with 5 and work up to whatever you are comfortable with, whether 20 or 50.

23. Bicycle

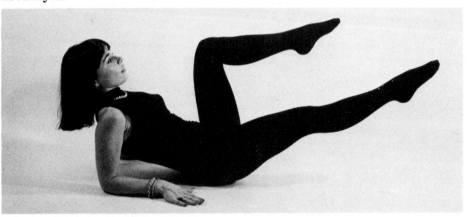

Sit on the floor and lean back on your elbows and forearms. Raise your legs, moving them in a circular motion as if you were pedaling a bicycle. As you bring one leg up over your chest, your other leg should extend straight out. At no time during this exercise should either of your legs touch the floor. Repeat this 16 times.

24. On elbows—knees to chest, straighten, and circle

As in the previous exercise, lean back on your elbows and forearms and bend your knees up over your chest. Release and straighten your legs, straight up, then slowly separate them. As they separate, they will lower, forming a circle in the air. The legs should be brought back together about 4 to 6 inches off the floor and held in that position for 3 seconds. Repeat the exercise 4 times. Each week you may add an additional rotation, but stop if you feel pain in your lower back at any time. Do this exercise a few weeks after you have begun the program, when your muscles are stronger and your body is in better shape. (Illustrations on opposite page.)

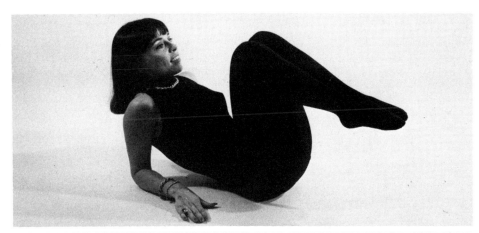

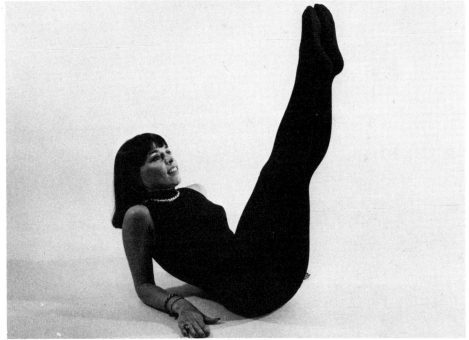

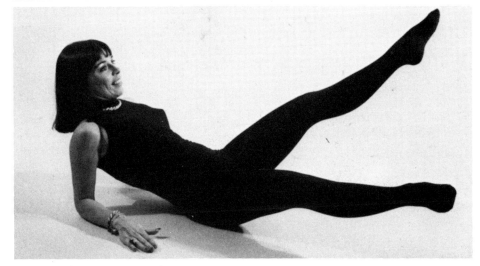

25. Standing—pelvic tilt

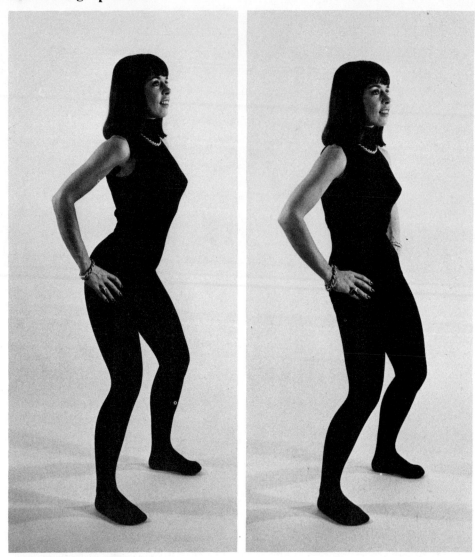

Place your feet apart and bend your knees slightly, with hands either on thighs or hips. Without moving your shoulders, push your buttocks out, then draw them under and tighten your abdominals. Do this 8 to 16 times, being careful not to move your legs or shoulders.

RECTUS ABDOMINUS

26. Hanging leg-lifts

Take hold of a bar placed well above your head. Keeping your legs straight, raise your feet off the ground and lift your legs in front of you as high as they will go. Hold your legs in the air for 4 seconds, then slowly return your feet to the floor. Repeat 4 to 6 times. In the beginning, don't worry if you can't raise your feet very high; with repetition, eventually you will be able to raise them nearly to the level of your stomach.

34

1. Back flat—leg-lower

This exercise is essential for lower-back strength, and, though it requires considerable effort and is slow in showing progress, it is one of the most important in the program. For illustration, see page 15.

Lie supine. Bring your knees up over your chest and then straighten your legs so that they form a 90-degree angle with your torso and the floor. Keeping the small of your back pressed firmly against the floor, slowly lower your legs. Be very careful to lower them only as far as you can, without allowing your back to rise off the floor. If you feel your back rising, you have lowered your legs too far. When you reach that point, hold the position for 4 seconds, then release by bending your knees over your chest. Rest and repeat 4 times. Never lower your legs all the way down to the floor, that will cause back strain. Be sure you go only as far as you can while keeping your back *flat*.

27. Back—arch and flatten

Lie supine. Bend knees to a 90-degree angle and place feet flat on the floor. Keeping your upper back and bottom on the floor, gently arch your lower back. Then flatten it, pressing it gently against the floor. Hold this position for 4 seconds and repeat the entire exercise 6 times.

GLUTEAL MUSCLE

28. Prone—tighten and release

Lie in a prone position, resting your forehead or your chin on folded arms. Tighten your abdominals, buttock muscles, inner thighs, and vaginal muscles. Hold the contractions for 4 seconds, then release. Repeat 6 times.

7. Donkey-kick—knee-to-nose

Get down on your hands and knees, keeping your arms straight. Bring your right knee up under your body. Try to touch your nose by bringing your face down to meet your knee. Then kick your leg out behind you, raising it as high as you can while lifting your head. Repeat 6 times, then change legs.

6. Prone—leg-lifts

Lie prone, resting your chin on your folded arms. Keeping your hipbones on the floor, raise your right leg without bending the knee. Hold leg in the air for 2 seconds, then lower it. Raise your left leg in the same manner. Repeat 16 times.

HAMSTRING

29. Sitting—side-to-side bounce, chin-to-toe, ear-to-knee

(a) Sit with your legs moderately wide apart and out straight. With both hands, hold your right knee and flex your right foot, stretching the calves and the backs of the thighs, including the tendons. Keeping your head and chin up, push your torso forward, then back, and pretend to touch your toes with 35

(cont'd)

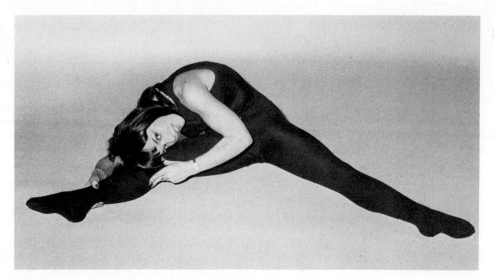

your indomitable chin. After 8 bounces, shift to the other leg, always keeping your chin, if not your spirits, up.

(b) Remain in the original position of the previous exercise. Instead of leading with your chin, try to touch your ear to your knee without bending the knee. Do it eight times, then reverse legs. This exercise will increase your flexibility.

9. Sitting—forward bounce, legs straight, feet together

Sit on the floor with your legs straight out in front of you and your feet together. Hold your legs, pull your torso forward, and then release it backward. You should feel a stretching in the backs of your legs. Bounce forward and back 16 times with your toes pointed, then flex your feet so that your toes point toward the ceiling and bounce 16 times.

8. Standing—forward bounce

Stand with feet apart, legs straight, and hands clasped behind you. Bounce forward, bending at the hips, as low as you can without bending your knees. Keeping your arms straight, bring your hands up behind you as you bounce forward. Bounce 8 times forward, then 8 times over the right leg, 8 times forward, 8 times over the left leg, and, finally, 8 times forward again. Be sure to keep your legs straight.

30. Standing—toes on book, heel lower

Stand with feet together and the balls of the feet resting on the edge of a thick book (phone books are great). Slowly lower your heels to the floor, then raise yourself onto the balls of your feet again, tightening your abdominals and buttock muscles in order to maintain your balance. Raise and lower your heels 16 times.

QUADRICEPS FEMORIS

31. Half knee-bend, heel down

Stand with feet together and arms outstretched straight in front of you.

Bend your knees as if going into a deep knee-bend, but go only halfway down. Your heels should remain flat on the floor. Do 16 times.

32. Side-to-side knee-bend

Stand with feet apart and arms at sides. Bend your left knee, leaning your weight on your left leg, keeping your right leg straight. Change sides, bending your right leg, keeping your left leg straight. Do 16 times.

33. Walk up-and-down stairs

Walk up and down a flight of stairs as many times as you can without discomfort.

34. On elbow—leg-lift

Lie on one side of your body and raise your torso off the floor by propping yourself up on an elbow, using forearm and hip for support. Lift your upper leg, like half of a scissors, up and down 6 times, keeping your toes pointed. Repeat 6 times with a flexed foot, being sure to keep your torso straight. Change sides and do it 12 more times.

35. On side—under leg-lift

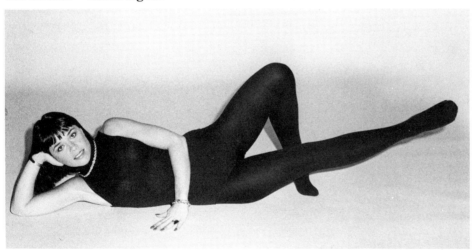

Lie on your right side, resting your head on your right hand to cushion your head from the floor. Bend your left leg, placing your left foot behind your right knee. Lift your right leg as far as you can, then lower it. Do this 6 times with toes pointed and 6 times with foot flexed; then change sides and repeat, raising left foot and bending right leg.

CALVES

36. Heel-up

Stand with feet together and place hands at your sides. Go up on the ball and toes of your right foot to raise the right heel while leaning your weight on your left leg. Alternate from right foot to left foot, holding each position to a count of 3, and repeat alternation 16 times.

37. Toe flex and curl

Stand with feet together. Curl your toes under as if trying to pick up a pencil with them; hold the position for 2 seconds. Uncurl your toes and pull them up toward your body; hold the position for 2 seconds. Repeat 8 times.

38. On toes—half knee-bend

Keeping your feet together, raise up on your toes. Slowly bend your knees, until you are in a half–knee-bend position; hold it for 4 seconds, then return to original position. Repeat 10 times.

3

The Body Shop

Each part of the human body should be kept in optimum working condition. Some parts may require greater attention than others, but the entire body will benefit from a complete exercise program. One's body is not altogether different from a car, for both require repeated servicings and considerate driving in order to be kept in optimum running condition.

The Weakest Links

From our own experience as teachers, we have encouraged students of all ages to develop the entire body, to keep it in optimum working condition.

If weak abdominals cause the stomach to slope, a strain begins to plague the lower back which will eventually result in pain. For example, there is no point in jogging without doing sit-ups. There is no easy way to fitness; it requires motivation, determination, and thirty minutes of your time every day.

From the concept of complete fitness, we have developed a top-to-toe, five-minute exercise routine. It is not a substitute for a complete workout; it is a handy supplement to fall back on when you are really short of time. The routine can be done by yourself or with a partner, and you will find it in detail at the conclusion of this chapter.

From the Beginning Now

We have emphasized the importance of self-evaluation, and you must realize that without honesty it is difficult to reach your peak of fitness. You've examined your body in a mirror and entered your measurements on the chart, so now you know what you like about yourself and what you intend to change. But before we go on, you need to know more about the most noticeable areas of your body.

Feet First

Feet are not strenuously exercised, not even by those who make wine from grapes. However, feet are of inestimable importance in providing essen- 39 tial balance, while carrying one through exercises as well as sports. You should not wear shoes which are too tight and cramp the toes. Grace, as well as balance while walking and running, comes from the toes. A perfect example is the idealized Indian moving noiselessly, like the wind, through woods and fields. Such noble savages did not float on air; rather, they went on bare feet or worse loose-fitting moccasins. In all of our exercise classes, each student goes barefoot.

Achilles Was No Heel

As ice skaters, skiers, and tennis players well know, ankles are as important to their quick movements as are stick shifts to racing car drivers. In both cases, movements must not only be swift, but they must be executed with such skill that there is barely room for error. If one has fat ankles, then one must diet as well as exercise. Fat gets in the way of quick movement. Exercise, by itself, will not trim ankles; however, exercise will stretch the Achilles tendon as well as limber up the entire foot area.

Our exercises will help keep your ankles lithe and limber. Furthermore, that noblest of tendons will be the beginning of your strength, flexibility, and endurance.

The Calves Jumped Over the Moon

Most people who spend their days sitting and their nights sleeping have tightly contracted calf muscles. Such people rarely, if ever, do much walking, never mind jogging. Their calf muscles are so tight, so contracted that if they tried a basic broad-jump, their subsequent pain would make them feel as if they had tried to jump over the moon.

As with the Achilles tendon, the calf muscles should be stretched, limbered, and without excess fat. Olympic runners have ideal legs, without an extra ounce of fat.

If you wish to commence a daily program of jogging, first do some simple stretching exercises. They will prevent subsequent pain and make jogging easier. The calf muscle benefits as much from stretching exercises as it does from exercises designed to increase strength. In fact, the same exercises will trim down thick calves, or build up skinny ones, adding a sensuous curve to an undistinguished line.

Beauty Is in the Thigh of the Beholder

Women tend to suffer more from heavy thighs than men, for women tend to develop inordinate wads of cellulite on their thighs. We devote a separate chapter to cellulite, in which we discuss special cellulite exercises, prescribe massages, and offer diet suggestions.

The ideal thigh should be comprised of long, elegant muscles. On both men and women, lean strong legs are a sign of agility, strength, and endurance. And, of course, they are extremely attractive. Unfortunately, many women are under the misapprehension that any kind of exercise will give them big, bulky legs. Not so. In fact, such legs are invariably a sign of advancing obesity as well as long periods of inactivity. Women who walk a great deal usually have slim, graceful legs. We advise you to walk whenever you have the time.

Hip, Hip Hooray!

The shape of a woman's hips determines the overall shape of her body, whether she is coming or going. Hips that are generous, without being fat, are the basis for what is commonly known as an hour-glass figure. Other women are as slim as models and seem to have no hips to speak of. Neither figure type is an ideal, but it is important, at least from an aesthetic point of view, that a woman's hips fit the rest of her figure.

Our hipstercises can help trim down bulky hips while building up small ones. Overabundant hips are a more commonplace problem, and they require not only exercise, but dieting and massage. Cellulite is often part of the problem, affecting buttocks, hips, and thighs. The hipstercises are at the conclusion of this chapter, while the dieting and massage information can be found in the chapter that deals with cellulite.

Bottoms Up

If you overeat and underexercise, you are likely to have a large, saggy, dimpled bottom. There may be no such item as a perfectly shaped bottom, but many shapes can and should be improved. The largest and certainly the most obvious muscle of all is found in the bottom, and it is the gluteus maximus. Others are the gluteus medius and gluteus minimous. When they receive the proper isometric and isotonic exercises, they will be hard, smooth, and shapely.

Waist Not, Want Not

As the summer of your life passes, with neither proper exercise nor proper diet, you may unhappily notice that your stomach is no longer flat and sexy. But if you really want a stomach as flat as a mythical teen-ager's, you haven't set an insurmountable goal. First, you have to be willing to consume only as many calories as you will burn up. Second, you must practice pulling in your stomach and tightening your abdominals. That will begin to add tone to those formerly underworked muscles. Though this is only an isometric exercise, it should be an integral part of any program designed to flatten your stomach. Third, our variety of sit-ups, plus our specially designed waistercises, will help to narrow your waist.

And both men and women should realize that girdles, or other similar devices, are no substitute for a strong stomach. A girdle simply pushes all of the abdominal organs into an uncomfortable proximity.

Backed into a Corner

We repeat, if the abdominals are weak, the lower-back muscles have to work overtime, resulting in pain that comes from the constant tension of trying to support the abdominals. Posture will suffer, and lower-back pain will be the result.

If you now suffer from lower-back pain, see a back specialist who can prescribe exercises that will relieve the pain and restore the strength in your back. If you have no back pain, we strongly suggest that you do the back exercises at the conclusion of this chapter as preventive medicine.

Breasts: The Bare Truth

For many women, the size and shape of their breasts will always be a source of self-conscious doubt. For some women, their breasts are too large and often too pendulous. For others, their breasts are embarrassingly small, and the expression "your cup runneth over" inspires envy.

In our experience in teaching gymnastics to teen-age girls, we have noticed that all of them develop breasts in superb proportion to the rest of their bodies. The reason for that is simple: They are exercising their entire bodies while building up strong pectoral muscles. Those muscles push out small breasts, making the mammary gland seem larger than it actually is. An adult woman can easily experience the same development; she need only strengthen her pectorals, using the isometric and isotonic exercises provided in this chapter.

If you have breasts that are too pendulous, you may only have to lose weight. An overweight woman is very likely to develop unhealthful layers of fat on her mammary glands; the weight of that fat will cause the entire breast to sag, in turn straining the pectoral muscles so that they are unable to provide optimum support.

Pectoral power is absolutely essential for any man who wishes to be completely fit. Without strong pectorals, the arms would lack pushing power to play an effective game of tennis, to shoot a few baskets, to swim with speed and endurance. Strong pectorals keep the layers of skin covering the chest from becoming loose and saggy. A soft, flabby chest is a sure sign of laziness and oncoming obesity; as one gets older, it can only get worse.

Shoulders Back Soldiers

Your shoulders should be held back, not only because you will have a sculptured line, but because the pectoral muscles will be properly stretched. Correctly and comfortably held shoulders do, indeed, aid good posture, helping to prevent upper-and-lower-back pain. Of course, one need not march around the living room like a raw recruit, nor need one do anything unnatural with one's body. And don't *throw* your shoulders back, for you might experience sudden and excruciating pain.

Graceful and well-placed shoulders develop from strong deltoid muscles, which aid in sports and exercise as well as adding symmetrical lines to the body.

Armed for Life

Arms are more important than most people realize; they are symbols of health and strength. The best condition of your arms is one of smooth muscularity without a drop of fat. Unfortunately, many men and women have arms heavy with fat and cellulite, a condition which can be alleviated and often entirely eliminated.

On Face Value

If you are in excellent shape, eat a well-balanced diet, and get adequate amounts of sleep, then your face will reveal the high value placed on the condition of your body.

An overtired body has a face which looks overtired, if not haggard. If you are nervous and tense, your face will be marked by signs of tension and nervousness. If your body is either too skinny or too fat, your face will not hide the weight.

Yet you can affect the appearance of your countenance by exercising, by dieting, and by doing our special face-saving exercises.

However, one should know that facial exercises have absolutely no effect on wrinkles. They develop because the skin dries out and that process may be accelerated by the reduction of the oxygen-carrying capacity of the blood vessels. Smoking, for instance, causes blood vessels to contract, so that they deliver insufficient quantities of oxygen to the skin. Heavy smokers have faces which are as lined as road maps.

Since voluntary muscles are utilized to manipulate facial expressions, it is important to know that by exercising those muscles you can insure a smooth, firm face. The muscles around the mouth and cheeks, especially, can easily be manipulated and exercised, and their well-toned appearance will give an air of youthfulness.

The Exorcist: Ridding Yourself of Devilish Aches and Pains

Those muscles which commonly experience numerous aches and pains are crying out for the attention of a good exercise program. When properly exercised, muscles can withstand certain sudden strains far better than muscles which are inadequately exercised.

Most people do not realize that they have kept their muscles in a contracted position for a significant period of time, thus limiting the circulation of blood to those muscles. The result, quite often, is a muscle spasm which can be as debilitating as it is painful.

This can develop in any of the voluntary muscles, not just the ones found in the legs. We have seen many people suffering from muscle spasms in their shoulders, necks, upper and lower backs, as well as stomachs. Backs are a particularly vulnerable area. A contracted back muscle, one rarely exercised, can be the source of a serious problem and, once it develops, may need medical treatment. As such a condition worsens, it can develop into a "trigger point." The phrase refers to muscles that are hard and knotted, thus causing excruciating pain that can leave the body incapacitated.

As if insufficient exercise were not enough cause for pain, stress, and tension are further responsible for just as much pain. Many people keep tension bottled up and let it ferment. One of the best ways to release that tension is to exercise. Tense muscles are even more contracted than under-exercised muscles, but after they have been exercised, they are stretched and relaxed, ready for either pleasure or sleep.

Coffee Breaks; Exercise Builds

Most people believe that exercise should be done either in one's home or at an exercise studio. However, exercise can be done just about anyplace. After we were married and worked in offices, we closed our office doors for ten minutes in the morning and ten minutes in the afternoon. In complete privacy, we were able to do push-ups, sit-ups, stretching exercises, and even chin-ups. We installed portable chinning bars in our doorways so we could do pull-ups or let-downs whenever we felt like it. This proved to be so popular that we had to get chinning bars for our co-workers.

Sometime between breakfast and lunch, most people trot off to a coffee cart. Having chatted, most people then return to their desks where they sip their expensive cups of coffee and nibble at their fattening pieces of cake. They are usually unaware of what the coffee is doing to their hearts, and they prefer not to think about all the calories in their yummy cakes, which are converted into rolls of fat. You would be infinitely better off with a piece of fruit and a few minutes of exercise to firm and tone muscles going soft during a day of sitting.

Isometricks for Travelers

We recently wrote an article entitled "Nine Ways to Exercise in an Airplane," which was published in an inflight magazine.

Few people had realized they could exercise while flying; fewer still have realized they could also exercise in buses, cars, trains, taxis—and even in dirigibles. Since isometrics require neither much space nor apparatus, they are ideal for travelers. The muscles which are exercised are merely contracted, then released, and at times they are pressed against stationary objects. As isometrics are done unobtrusively, one need not feel self-conscious about attracting unwanted attention.

The simple activity itself can break up the monotony of a journey, even when one is strapped to a seat. The pleasant result is a sense of relaxation and a state free of fatigue and tension.

Washercise: Cleanliness Can Be Close to Fitness

A hot bath or a hot shower provides an environment conducive to exercise. There, one's tense, contracted muscles can pleasantly relax. In addition, in a tub of water the effects of gravity are hardly felt. Not only are muscles relaxed, but they feel almost weightless, and exercises become seemingly effortless. But while in the bath or shower don't attempt exercises that are so vigorous that they require a great deal of movement. More accidents occur in bathrooms, especially in tubs, than in any other place in the home. So be careful and use common sense.

The Five-Minute Dance Which Exercises the Entire Body

Exercises should be varied, if for no other reason than to avoid monotony. Suzy has developed a simple but delightful dance routine which only takes five minutes to perform but which exercises all the muscles in the body. It can be done with or without a partner. The routine is actually a series of warm-up exercises, but they should not be regarded as a substitute for a regular exercise routine. It is a supplementary activity, but on days when time is really limited, it is better than no exercise at all.

Choose one of your favorite tunes, something with an upbeat, and then just move to the music. Make sure the tempo is not so fast that you can't get in all the exercises. Each exercise provides a small workout for particular muscles or a body area; each movement naturally leads into a related movement, creating one graceful routine.

From the Bottom Up

FEET

39. Curl feet and flatten

Stand with your feet together and your arms at your sides. Shift your feet so that your weight is on the outsides of your feet and curl your toes under. Hold for 4 seconds, then return to a flatfooted stance. Do 8 times.

37. Toe flex and curl

Stand with your feet together and curl your toes under as if trying to pick up a pencil. Hold for 2 seconds. Uncurl your toes and pull them up toward your body. Hold for 2 seconds. Repeat 8 times.

40. Toe stretch and release

This exercise may be done while standing, sitting, or even lying down, but be sure your feet are bare. Stretch and separate your toes, holding this position for 4 seconds before releasing and relaxing your feet. Repeat 10 times for each foot. Then curl your toes under and hold this position for 2 seconds to release the tension in your foot. *Do not* continue the exercise if your foot cramps. Return to it later.

ACHILLES TENDON AND ANKLES

41. Sitting—foot circle

Sit in a chair. Cross your right leg over your left knee and relax. (You can do this exercise anywhere.) Move your dangling right foot 8 times in a clockwise circular motion, then 8 times counterclockwise. Repeat twice, then change legs. Switch again and do the series twice.

45

42. Sitting—foot flex and point

As in exercise 43, sit with your right leg crossed over your left knee. Flex your right foot, pulling your upper foot and toes up toward your body and hold for 4 seconds. Then point your entire foot and toes downward and hold for 4 seconds. Repeat 8 times, then change feet. Do 8 times with left foot and repeat entire series once more.

This exercise, as with exercise 43, may be done at any time and is soothing for sore and tired feet at the end of the day, for cold and stiff feet during or after skiing or skating, and for feet that receive little or no exercise.

30. Standing—toes on book, heel-lower

Stand with feet together, with the balls of the feet resting on the edge of a thick book (phone books are great). Slowly lower your heels to the floor; then raise yourself onto the balls of your feet again. Be sure to tighten your abdominals and buttock muscles to maintain your balance. Raise and lower your heels 16 times.

43. Knee wag

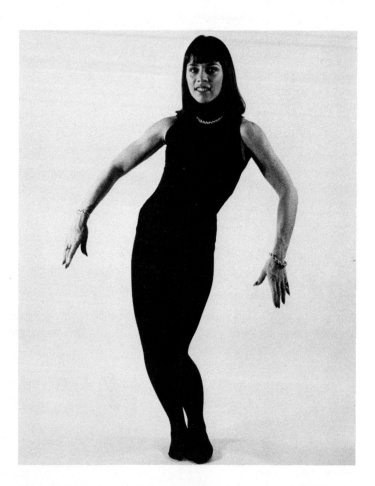

Stand with your feet and knees together; bend your knees slightly and lean on the outer part of your right foot and the inner part of your left one, and then sway your knees to the right. Alternate the direction of your sways, moving back and forth 16 times.

44. Snowplow knee-bend

Stand with your feet apart but turned inward as if you are pigeon-toed. Your knees and thighs should be touching, but your calves should be apart. Stand up, straightening your legs. Do 16 times.

45. Sitting—toe pointed against rope

Sit on the floor with legs stretched out in front of you. Place the middle of a rope or towel against the balls of your feet, while holding an end in each hand. Gently pull the rope or towel against your feet, creating pressure. While pulling, push your feet against the rope or towel until your feet point forward. Now release your feet and return to the original position with toes pointed up toward the ceiling and rope or towel resting gently against the balls of your feet. Repeat 6 times.

This exercise may also be done while sitting in a chair and stretching out one leg at a time. Place the rope against the foot that is raised and repeat 6 times with each foot.

46. Rope jump

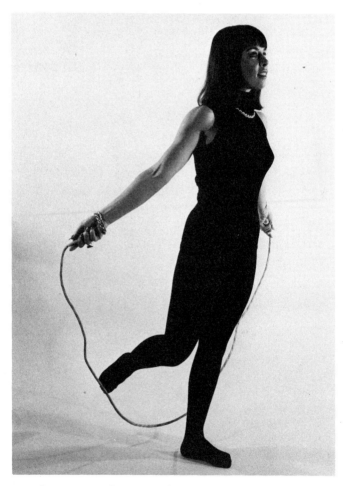

There are many ways to jump rope; however, here we shall only deal with two ways. (The length of the rope should be determined by your own height.) Hold an end in each hand and relax your arms at your sides. Two   47

(cont'd)

feet of the center of the rope should be resting on the floor. Less than that will cause you to miss jumps and perhaps trip and injure yourself.

A. *Feet together jump:* Starting with the rope resting behind your feet, which are together, swing the rope around and up, letting it pass over your head, then down onto the floor in front of your feet. As the rope hits the floor it should be pulled back toward you as you jump over it. As your coordination develops, you may add an extra jump between jumps over the rope. You may find it easier to take a big jump as the rope hits the floor and is pulled back toward your feet. Get a steady rhythm going and jump for about 30 seconds only. In time you may work up to 3 minutes, but never exceed either your stamina or your abilities of coordination.

B. *Step jump:* Start with the rope resting behind your feet, which are together, then swing the rope up and over your head, letting it land on the floor in front of your feet. As the rope hits the floor in front of you, pull it back toward your feet and hop over it with your right foot. As you bring the rope back up over your head, step onto your left foot. Continue hopping over the rope with your right foot and stepping onto your left foot. Repeat 10 times and change feet. Don't overdo. After a few weeks, you will have no trouble alternating from your right foot to your left foot, increasing your hops, but start slowly and work up to it. This exercise is good for your calves and your heart, and ten minutes of it is equal to 30 minutes of jogging.

THIGHS

47. On elbows—frog kick

Sit on the floor and lean back on your elbows and forearms. Bend your legs at the knees and bring your knees over your chest. Slowly separate your knees and put the soles of your feet together. Stretch your legs and feet apart, straightening out your legs like open scissor blades. Then close those scissors and bring your legs and ankles together again about 6 to 8 inches from the floor. Hold for 2 seconds. Return to the position with your legs bent over your chest. Do 8 times, but stop if you experience any strain or pain in your lower back.

48. On elbows—scissors crossover

As in the previous exercise, sit on the floor and lean back on your elbows

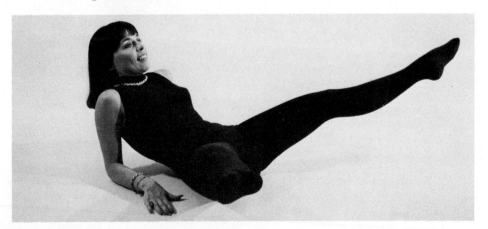

and forearms with your legs apart. Raise your legs off the floor and flex your feet, turning your toes outward. Then turn your toes inward, facing each other, and cross your left leg over your right. From the completed crossover position, turn your feet outward and move your legs into the spread position again. Keep straightened legs off the floor and reverse the order, passing your right foot over your left. Do 8 times; stop if you experience any lower-back pain or strain.

34. On elbow—leg-lift

Lie on one side of your body; raise your torso off the floor by propping yourself on an elbow, using your forearm and hip for additional support. Lift your upper leg, like half of a scissors, up and down 6 times, keeping your toes pointed. Repeat 6 times with a flexed foot. Be sure to keep your torso straight. Change sides and repeat 6 times.

35. On side—under leg-lift

Lie on your right side, resting your head on your right bicep to cushion your head from the floor. Bend your left leg placing your left foot behind your right knee. Lift your straight right leg as far as you can; then lower it. Do 6 times with toes pointed and 6 times with foot flexed. Change sides and repeat, raising left foot and bending right leg.

49. Infinity leg-swing

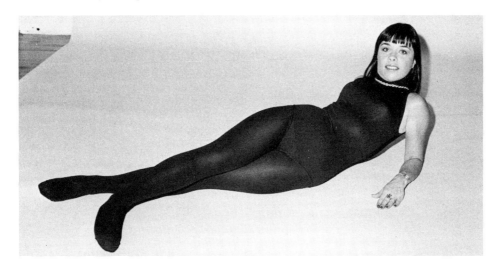

Sit on the floor, lean back on your elbows and forearms, and stretch your legs out in front of you. Flex your right foot and lift it, turning it to the left. Cross it over your left leg until you can place your right large toe just beyond your left leg. Reverse the motion, bring your right foot back, turning the entire foot to the right. Repeat 6 times and change legs. Do 6 with left leg.

HIPS

50. Sitting, L position—leg-lifts

Sit on the floor with your left leg bent at the knee, your left calf crossing in front of your crotch and your left foot pointed toward your right leg. Bend 49

(cont'd)

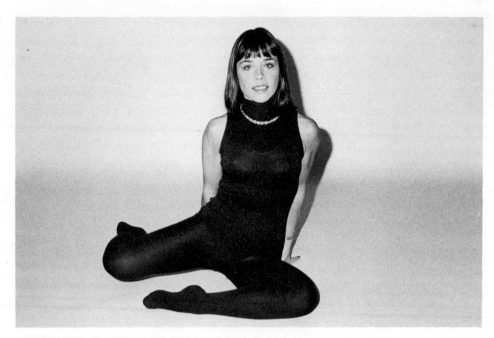

your right leg at your side, your right calf next to but not touching your right buttock, and your right foot pointing back. Rest your palms on the floor behind you, but do not place your weight on them; they are for balance only. Keeping your body straight and your right leg bent, raise and lower your right leg 12 times. Reverse the position of your legs, crossing your right leg in front of you and bending your left leg to your left side. Raise and lower your left leg 12 times. Repeat series twice.

51. Sitting, L position—leg-lift and stretch

Sit as in exercise 50 with left leg bent and crossed in front of you and right leg bent out to your right side. Keep your body facing forward and rest

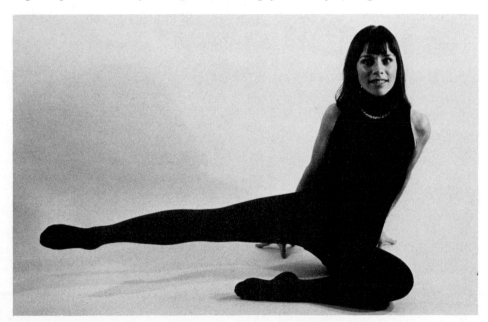

on your palms which are behind you. Raise your right leg, being sure it remains out to the side and does not move forward. When the entire leg is 3 to 6 inches off the floor, straighten leg out to the side, hold for 3 seconds and return it to a bent-knee position. Lower your leg to the floor. Repeat 6 times, being sure to hold your torso in an upright position. Reverse positions, crossing your right leg in front of you and bending your left leg out to the side. Repeat exercise 6 times with your left leg. Do series twice.

52. On hands and knees—Leg-stretch

Get down on your hands and knees. Keeping your right leg bent in an L position, raise it as high as you can to your right side with your weight resting evenly on your flat palms. Stretch your right leg out to the side as far as you can and feel the muscles stretching outward. Hold this position for 2 seconds

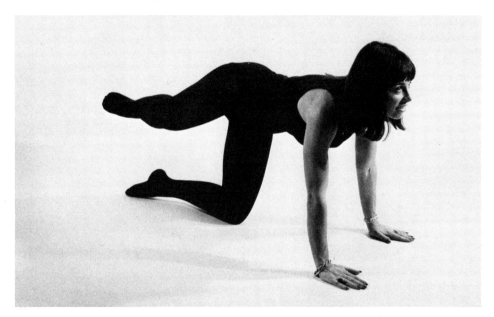

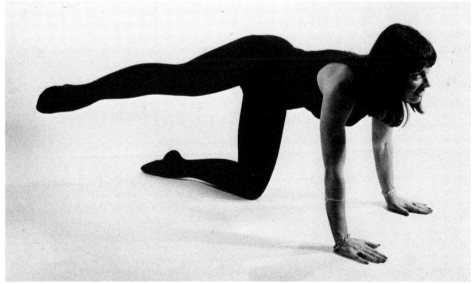

51

(cont'd)

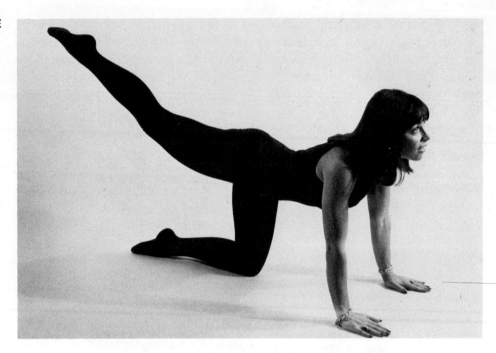

and release, bending your right leg in again but keeping it in the air. Swing your right leg out behind you, stretching it straight and slightly upward, keeping your right hip no higher than your left hip. Release this backward stretched position by bending your right knee and returning it to the original raised position at your right side. (Be sure your leg is raised as high as possible in the L position.) Then return your knee to the floor. Reverse legs and repeat entire exercise with left leg. Do series 4 times. Remember that when leg is raised to the side, hip should be lifted; when leg is stretched behind you, hip should be lowered.

53. Hip-lift

Stand with your feet slightly apart and arms at a 45-degree angle from your body. Raise your right hip and move it forward slightly. You will be raising your right heel as your right foot goes up on its toes. Your hip should be turned slightly inward, as if you were trying to glance at your right buttock without the aid of a mirror. Lower your hip and place your foot flat on the floor again. Repeat 6 times. Reverse legs and do the exercise 6 times with your left hip.

BOTTOM

54. Standing—leg-swing

Stand straight, using your left hand to balance yourself by placing it on the back of a chair, couch, or counter. Keep your left leg perfectly straight, and kick the air in front of you with your right leg. Bring it up as high as you can, and then swing it backward up behind yourself. Keep your kicking foot facing forward and your leg straight. Swing leg forward and back 8 times, then reverse legs. Turn around and place your right hand on whatever you are using for balance while your left leg kicks forward and back.

55. Standing—donkey-kick

Stand with feet slightly apart and legs straight. Place the palms of both hands on the floor about three feet in front of you, leaning weight equally on hands and feet. Keeping your arms and your left leg straight, bring your right knee up under your body and touch it to your nose while lowering your head. Kick your right leg out behind you, straightening and lifting it as high as you can while lifting your head. Repeat 8 times and change legs. It's easy to lose your balance, so take your time. If you start to fall over, then you're moving too fast. Tighten your abdominals; this will help you maintain your balance.

56. Prone—leg-lift, feet apart

Lie on your stomach, resting your chin on your folded arms. Keep your legs straight and feet 3 feet apart, with your hipbones on the floor. Alternate, lifting first one leg, holding it for 4 seconds, then the other leg. Repeat 16 times.

57. On knees—figure 8

Get down on your hands and knees and keep your arms straight. With your left knee bent and your weight resting evenly on your hands and left knee, straighten your right leg out to your right side. Lift your right foot off the floor, swinging the leg up and over the left foot. Bring the right foot to rest behind and to the left of your left foot. Then raise your right leg in an arc again, returning your right foot to its original position. Repeat 8 times; then reverse legs.

WAIST

58. Holding hands— side-to-side bounce

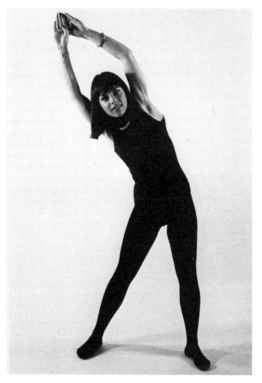

Stand with feet apart and stretch your arms upward, clasping your hands together above your head. From your waist, arc your body to the right with- 53

(cont'd)

out turning it. Bounce your torso 4 times to the side over your right leg. Change direction, curving your body to the left, and bounce 4 more times. As you bounce, be sure to stretch your arms.

59. Getting off the rack

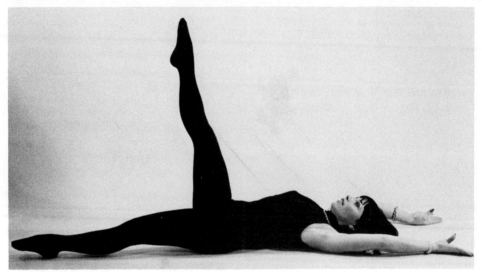

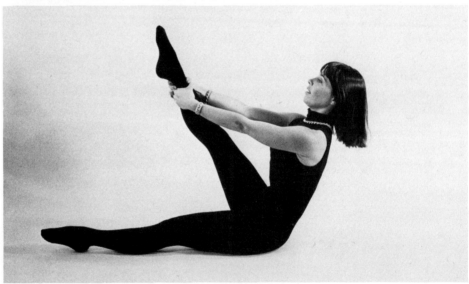

Lie supine with your arms and legs outstretched. Raise your right leg straight up into the air. In one motion, swing your arms up, sit up, and grab your right ankle with both hands. If you cannot reach your ankle without bending your knee, then grab your calf. Straighten your back by arching your lower back and pulling your stomach and chest toward your uplifted leg. Hold for 3 seconds, then let go and gently return to the original supine position. Do 8 times and reverse legs.

60. Elbow snap

Standing with legs apart, hold your arms at shoulder height, but bend them at the elbows. Now turn your torso twice to the right, twice to the left.

While twisting your torso, you should keep your legs stationary and not move your hips. Twist 16 times in each direction.

LOWER BACK

1. Back flat—leg-lower

This exercise is essential for lower-back strength. If you feel pain in your lower back, make sure you are doing it correctly. This exercise often seems to require more effort than it's worth, but though it's slow to show results, it's one of the most important. See page 15 for illustration.

Lie supine. Bring your knees up over your chest and straighten your legs so that they form a 90-degree angle with your torso and the floor. Keeping the small of your back pressed firmly against the floor, slowly lower your legs. Be careful to lower them only as far as you can without your back rising off the floor. (If you feel your back rising, you have lowered your legs too far.) When you reach that point, hold the position for 4 seconds; then release by bending your knees over your chest. Rest and repeat 4 times. *Never* lower your legs all the way to the floor, that will cause back strain. Be sure to go *only* as far as you can while keeping your back flat.

27. Back—arch and flatten

Lie supine. Bend your knees to a 90-degree angle with feet flat on the floor. Keeping your upper back and bottom on the floor, gently arch your lower back. Then flatten it, gently pressing it against the floor. Hold the flattened position for 4 seconds, and repeat the exercise 6 times.

61. The metronome

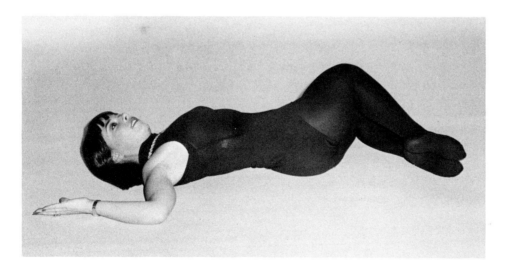

Lie supine. Raise your legs, bending your knees up over your chest. Press the small of your back against the floor, and slowly lower your bent legs to the left, trying to keep both shoulders on the floor. Lift your bent legs off the floor, bringing them up over your chest again while pressing the small of your back against the floor. Slowly lower your legs to the right side. Repeat 16 times.

62. Sitting—back-push and release

Sit straight in a chair with your knees bent and feet flat on the floor. Rest your arms on the arms of the chair, with your back supported by the back of the chair. Tighten your abdominal muscles and slowly press the lower part of your back against your chair. Hold this position for 4 seconds; then relax your stomach and back muscles. Repeat 6 to 8 times.

63. The feline

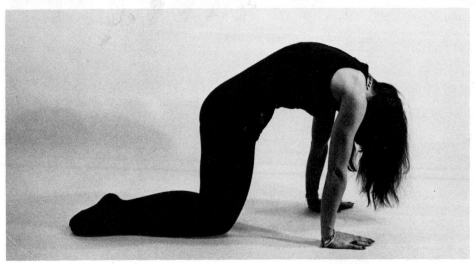

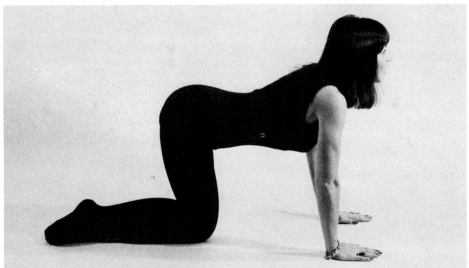

Get down on your hands and knees. Slowly lower your head and round your back, lifting it upward while you suck in your stomach. Hold for 3 seconds, then raise your head and slowly lower your back, letting it sag in the middle. Repeat 8 times.

UPPER BACK

64. Prone—double arm-lifts

Lie prone with your chin on the floor and your arms stretched out straight in front of you, your feet anchored under something secure. Raise both straight arms, your head, and your chest off the floor as high as you can. Hold this position for 4 seconds; then return to your original position for 4 more seconds. Repeat 8 times.

65. Pushing marbles with your nose

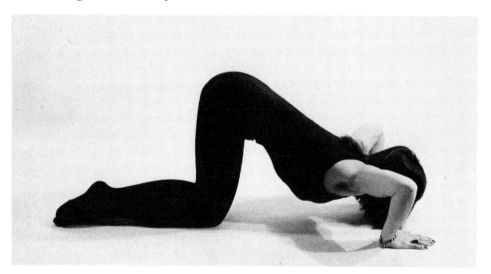

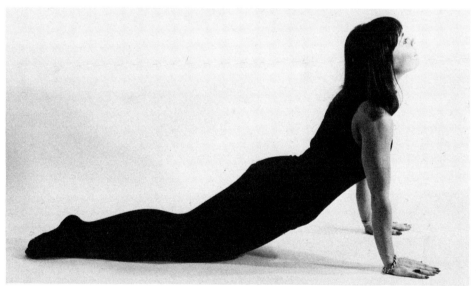

Get down on your hands and knees and stretch your arms out as far as you can in front of you, resting your bottom on your heels. Move your torso forward, keeping your head close to the floor as if pushing a marble with your nose. Your head will travel past your arms which should be bent at the elbows. After your nose has gone as far as possible, raise your head and straighten your arms, pushing your entire torso upward. Return to the original position with your bottom resting on your heels, and repeat the exercise 4 times.

66. On slant board, prone—weighted butterfly

Lie prone on a slant board, with your head at the raised end, and stretch your arms out onto the floor. Keep them at right angles to your body. Grasp 3-pound weights in each hand and, holding arms straight, raise and lower them like the wings of a butterfly. Repeat 8 times and rest. If you do not have a slant board, an ironing board will serve the same purpose. Put books or blocks which are 6 to 10 inches high, beneath one end, and rest your head on that raised end. Before beginning the exercise, test the board for sturdiness and balance.

67. Sitting—curl-up and stretch

Sit with your knees bent and your feet on the floor. Keeping your legs together, clasp them with encircling hands and tuck your head down as you round your back and tighten you abdominals. Hold for 4 seconds, and do not tighten your shoulders. Release your legs and place your hands on the floor

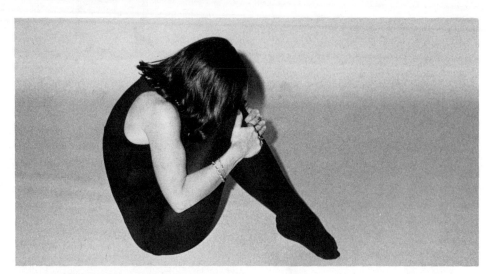

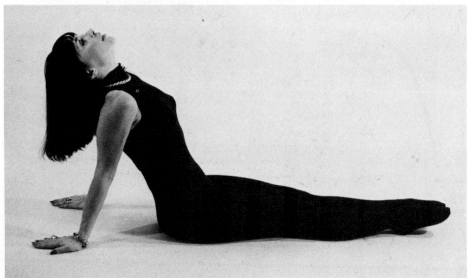

behind you. Thrust your chest up into the air, arching your back and straightening your legs. Hold for 4 seconds without lifting your buttocks from the floor. Repeat series 8 times.

68. Dowel—arm-swing

Stand with feet apart and hold the 3-foot dowel at each end in front of your chest. The dowel should be horizontal with the floor. Keeping your arms at shoulder height, swing from side to side, following the motion of your arms with your head. Keep your hips and thighs stationary and do 16 times.

69. Sitting—side push-ups to straight-leg crab

Sit on the floor with your feet apart and legs straight out. Lean over to your right side, placing both hands on the floor in line with your shoulders. Lower your upper torso to the floor and then push away, sitting up straight. Lean forward to touch your toes, keeping legs straight. Then put your hands on the floor behind you and push your buttocks upward, lifting your hips off the floor as high as you can and hold for 4 seconds. (Illustrations continued on page 60.) Return to the sitting position and repeat exercise, this time moving to your left side. Repeat series 8 times.

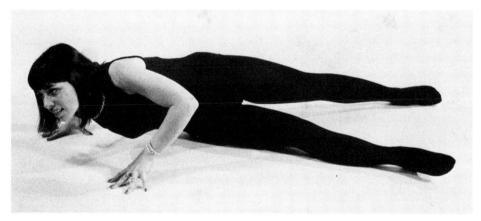

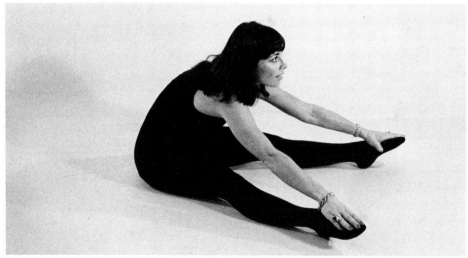

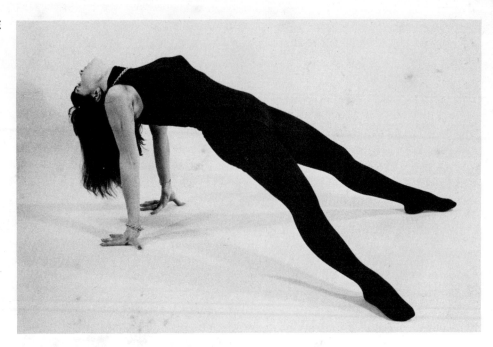

70. With towel—pull and release

Stand with your feet apart. Grasp a small towel by the corners and raise your bent arms to shoulder height. Pull the towel taut from opposite ends and hold for 4 seconds before releasing. Repeat 12 times.

71. With chest expander—pull and release (for men)

Hold a chest expander across your chest while standing with feet apart. Pull outward as far as you can and hold for 4 seconds, then release. Repeat 10 times without strain and try to work up to 30, adding 5 or 6 each week.

72. On slant board, supine—weighted butterfly

Lie supine on a slant board (or raised ironing board) with your head at the higher end and your arms stretched out at right angles from your body,

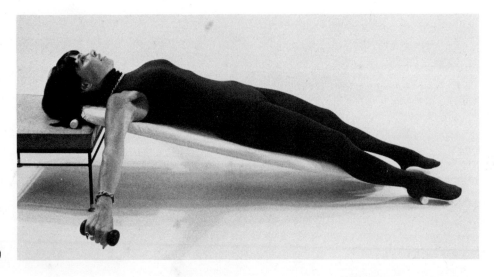

hanging to the floor. Grasp a 3-pound weight in each hand and, with arms THE BODY SHOP straight, raise your hands off the floor to meet in the air above your chest. Slowly lower your arms and rest your hands on the floor again. Repeat 8 times.

SHOULDERS

13B. The shrug

Standing with feet together and arms at your sides, try to raise your shoulders up to your ears. Lower your shoulders and lift your head, stretching your neck. Repeat 16 times.

73. Shoulder rotate

Stand with your feet apart and arms raised at your sides at shoulder height. Turn your right hand and arm under, thus turning your right shoulder forward. At the same time, turn your left hand and arm backward, turning your left shoulder back. Then change direction of both arms, turning left hand down and right hand up. Repeat 12 times.

74. Arm propeller

Stand with your feet apart and your arms at your sides. Swing one arm in a forward circular movement, up, back, and down. Don't be so vigorous that you twist a muscle. Do the exercise 8 times, then reverse the direction, after which repeat with other arm.

18. The back of my hand

This exercise can be done either with feet together or apart. Keep your left arm at your side and raise your right arm, bending it at the elbow. Place the back of your right hand against your right cheek and swing your arm, throwing your hand backward and away from your face until your arm is as straight as a backstroker's. Do the same with your left hand and arm, leaving your right at your side. Do this exercise 8 times with each arm.

75. Dowel—shoulder rotate

Hold a 3-foot-long dowel at each end in front of your thighs, keeping your arms straight. Slowly raise your straight arms in front of you, up above your head. Slowly continue moving your arms backward as far as you can, keeping your arms straight.

11. Shoulder twist

Stand with feet slightly apart, arms raised straight out to the sides at shoulder height. Stretching your arms outward, turn your palms up and then slowly forward, down, and up behind, allowing your shoulders to rotate forward. Hold the position for 4 seconds, and return to forward palms-up position for 4 seconds. Repeat 8 times.

76. Shoulder-twist circle

Stand with feet apart and arms stretched out at your sides at shoulder height. Turn your hands down and back, and outline circles in the air. This is effective for rotating the shoulder joint. Repeat 16 times forward and 16 times backward.

61

77. Head metronome

Stand or sit on a chair, but keep your back straight and your arms hanging at your sides. Lower your head to the right so that your right ear is above your right shoulder. Do *not* raise your shoulder. Straighten your neck, and then lower your head toward the left shoulder. Repeat 16 times.

78. Head twist

Keeping your back straight and your arms at your sides, stretch your neck upward without lifting your chin. Keeping your shoulders in place, slowly turn your head to the right until you are looking over your right shoulder, but go only as far as is comfortable. Slowly return to the center position, and then turn to the left, looking over your left shoulder. Return to the center and relax your back, shoulders, and neck. Straighten up again and repeat the entire series 8 times with slow, smooth movements.

79. Head back—open and close mouth

Slowly and gently let your head fall back so that your face is turned up toward the ceiling. Don't move the rest of your body. Open your mouth as wide as you can; then close it. You should feel a pulling sensation in your neck and under your chin. Repeat 8 times.

A FEW ON FLEXIBILITY

80. On hands and knees—forward leg-bounce and stretch

Get down on your hands and knees and stretch your right leg out behind you. Place your left foot flat on the floor to the left of your left hand. Supporting your weight on your left leg, lean your weight forward and backward. Repeat 8 times, then reverse legs.

81. Head down—knee-bend

Stand with your feet together and place your hands in front of your thighs. Bend your knees until your hands touch the floor on the outsides of your feet,

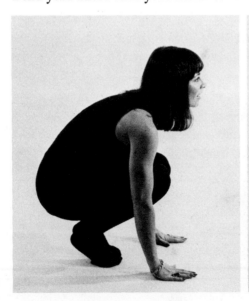
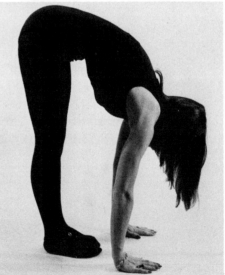

keeping your arms straight. With your hands on the floor, straighten your legs so that your bottom goes up. Hold for 3 seconds and then return to upright position. Do 8 times.

82. Up goes the leg

Recline on your right side, leaning on your right elbow and forearm. Bend your left leg at the knee, and bring the knee up toward your shoulder. With your left hand grab the inside of your left foot. Slowly straighten your left leg up as high as you can without pain and pull it toward your left shoulder 4 times, and release. Do 4 times, then reverse sides.

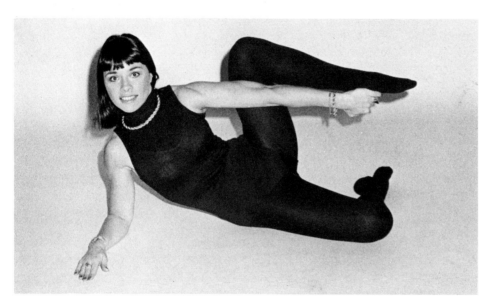

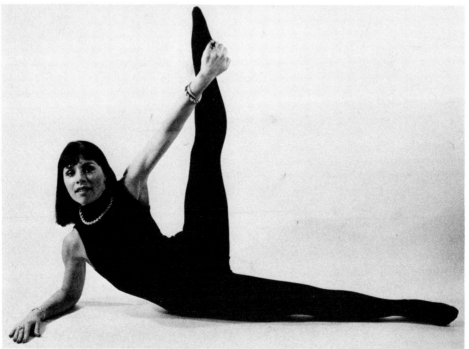

A Five-Minute Warm-Up to Loosen Tight Muscles and Make Exercising Pleasant and Beneficial

This routine should be done to music. We have chosen Paul Mauriat's "Love Is Blue," from his album *Blooming Hits*. The song is only two and a half minutes long, so it must be played twice to accompany the whole warm-up.

Below are seven new exercises not included in the previous pages. The remaining exercises have all been listed.

83. Feet apart—knee-bend

Stand with feet apart, arms slightly raised away from thighs and hips. Slowly bend your knees half way down, keeping your torso absolutely straight, and then stand up again.

84. Hip wag

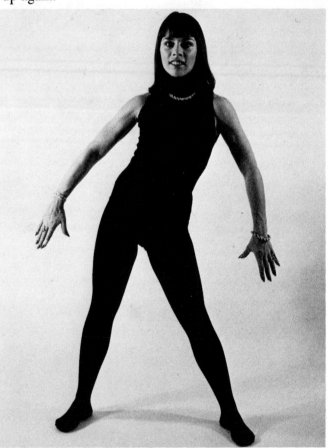

Stand with feet apart and arms slightly raised from your sides. Push your right hip to the right, leaning most of your weight onto your straight right leg and foot. Reverse direction to the left, and try to move to the rhythm of the music.

85. Airplane stretch and circle

Stand with feet apart, fingertips touching each other in front of your chest, elbows out at your sides and at shoulder height. Gently bring your elbows back behind you as far as they can go; then return to the original position. Straighten out your arms in front of you, then raise them straight up, backwards, then down, making a full circular motion. Return your arms to their first position—elbows bent and fingertips touching in front of your chest—and repeat entire exercise 8 times. Reverse circular motion and repeat 8 times.

86. Shoulder circle

Stand with feet slightly apart and arms at your sides. Tighten your abdominals and slowly push your shoulders forward. Lift your shoulders up to your ears and stretch them back as far as you can before lowering them to their original position. Repeat the forward circular motion 8 times; then reverse direction, circling your shoulders in a backward motion. Repeat 8 times.

87. Overhead arm-stretch

Stand with your feet together and stretch your arms up straight above your head. Bend your right leg at the knee, and stretch your right arm higher above your head as far as you can. Hold for 4 seconds. Release your right arm, still holding it above your head, and straighten your right leg. Bend your left leg at the knee, and stretch your left arm higher above your head as far as you can. Hold for 4 seconds. Release your left arm, still holding it above your head, and straighten your left leg. Repeat series 8 times.

88. Side-to-side leg-stretch and bounce

Stand with your feet apart and your hands clasped behind your buttocks. Keeping your left foot pointed forward, turn your right foot out to point

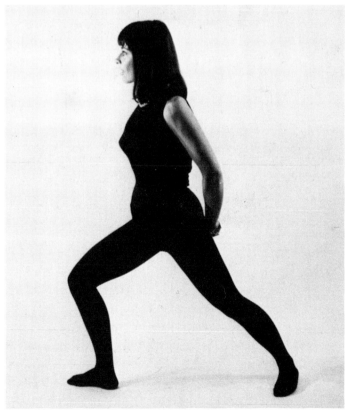

65

(cont'd)

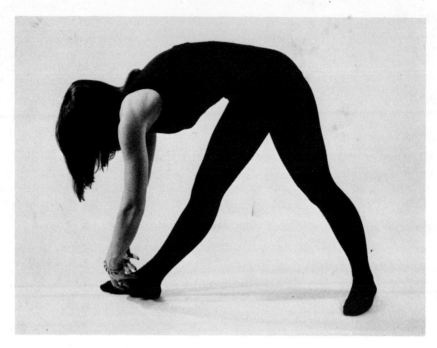

right, and turn your body until it faces right. Do 4 half knee-bends on your right leg while keeping your left leg straight. Straighten your right leg and do 4 forward bounces over your right leg, letting your hands hang down in front of you. Repeat series 4 times. Return your right foot to the original position, and turn your left foot to the left. Repeat exercise 4 times to the left.

89. Arm-swing

Stand with your feet apart and arms stretched out to the sides, level with your shoulders. Swing both arms, first to the left and then to the right, following the movement with your nose. Throughout, keep your hips from moving. Do 16 times.

To learn a routine, first listen to your music and familiarize yourself with it. Then look through the exercises to make sure you know what you will be doing. In the beginning, you'll need to keep checking the list for the order, but in a little while the music will carry you along naturally.

Exercises in Order

R1. Overhead arm stretch (12 times)
R2. The swim (16 times)
R3. Feet apart—knee-bend (1 time)
R4. Hip wag (8 single wags, 4 double wags)
R5. Feet apart—knee-bend (1 time)
R6. Side-to-side knee-bend (16 times)
R7. Feet apart—knee-bend (2 times)
R8. Airplane stretch (8 times)
R9. Heel-up (8 times feet separate, 4 times feet together)
R10. Overhead arm-stretch (8 times stretching once, 4 times stretching twice)

    R11. Overhead arm-stretch (12 times)
    R12. Standing—forward bounce (16 times)
    R13. Feet apart—knee-bend (1 time)
    R14. Side-to-side leg-stretch and bounce (8 times)
    R15. Feet apart—knee-bend (1 time)
    R16. Side-to-side leg-stretch and bounce (8 times)
    R17. Feet apart—knee-bend (2 times)
    R18. Airplane stretch and circle (4 times)
    R19. Shoulder circle (1 time)
    R20. Arm-swing (8 times)
    R21. Shoulders back and forth and the shrug (1 time)
    R22. Overhead arm-stretch (variation) (8 times bouncing once, 4 times bouncing twice)

Put the music on and start your routine.

R1. Overhead arm-stretch.

Stand with your feet together and stretch your arms straight up above your head. Bend your right leg at the knee, and stretch your right arm still higher above your head as hard and far as possible. Release your right arm, keeping it above your head, and straighten your right leg. Bend your left leg at the knee, and stretch your left arm above your head as hard and far as possible. Release your left arm, keeping it above your head, and straighten your left leg. Alternate arm-stretches 12 times, counting 3 sets of 4. 1234, 2234, 3234.

As you finish the third set of 4, place your feet apart and bend forward at the hips.

R2. The swim.

Stand with your feet apart and bend forward from the hips. Move your arms in a swimming motion, as if you were doing the crawl, making complete circular movements. Alternate arms 4 times while bending straight forward, 4 times bending over your right leg, 4 times bending over your left leg, and 4 times bending forward again. Count four sets of 4. 1234, 2234, 3234, 4234.

R3. Feet apart—knee-bend.

Stand with your feet apart, arms slightly raised away from your thighs and hips. Slowly bend your knees halfway, keeping your torso absolutely straight, and then stand up again. Do one knee-bend, count 1, 2.

R4. Hip-wag.

Stand with your feet apart and arms raised slightly from your sides. Push your hip to the right, leaning most of your weight onto your straight right leg. Reverse direction and do the same to the left. Alternate hips 4 times; then do a double hip-wag (bouncing twice) to the right once and then to the left once. Repeat single hip-wag to the left and right 4 times and double hip-wag to the right and left. Count four sets of 4.

R5. Feet apart—knee-bend.
    Do one knee-bend, count 1, 2.

R6. Side-to-side knee-bend.

Stand with your feet apart and arms at your sides. Bend your right knee, leaning your weight on your right leg, while keeping your left leg straight. Change sides, bending your left leg while keeping your right leg straight. Bend 4 times to the right and 4 times to the left; repeat 4 times to the right and 4 times to the left. Count 4 sets of 4.

R7. Feet apart—knee-bend.

Do two knee-bends, count 1, 2, 3, 4.

R8. Airplane stretch.

Standing with your feet apart, bring your arms up to shoulder height. Bend them at the elbows until your fingers touch in front of you. Quickly bring your elbows back as far as you can, then return them to the starting position. Straighten your arms out to the sides, still keeping them at shoulder height, and turn your palms upward. Return to the original position. Do 8, counting four sets of 4. Change position and stand with feet together, counting 1, 2.

R9. Heel-up.

Stand with your feet together and hands at your sides. Raise your right heel by going up on the ball and toes of your right foot, leaning your weight on your left leg. Alternate from right to left leg four times, counting to 4. Then raise both heels, counting to 2 while raising and to 2 while lowering. Do this twice, and then alternate right and left feet again 4 times, counting to 4. For entire series, count 4 sets of 4.

Do two half knee-bends, keeping feet together while slowly raising your arms straight above your head. Count to 4.

R10. Overhead arm-stretch (variation).

Stretch your right arm, then your left arm, again right arm, and then left arm, counting to 4. Then reach twice with the right arm, then twice with the left arm, and repeat, counting two sets of 4. Finally, repeat first set of arm-stretches, counting to 4. For the entire series, count 4 sets of 4.

Stand with your feet apart and slowly lower your arms to your sides as the music ends.

Repeat record, begin as before, with feet together and arms stretched straight above your head.

R11. Overhead arm-stretch.

Alternate 12 arm-stretches, counting 3 sets of 4.

R12. Standing—forward bounce.

Stand with your feet apart, legs straight, and hands clasped behind you. Bounce forward, bending at the hips, as low as you can without bending your knees. Keep your arms straight and bring your hands up behind you as you bounce forward. Bounce forward 4 times, over your right leg 4 times, over your left leg 4 times, and forward again 4 times. Count 4 sets of 4.

R13. Feet apart—knee-bend.

Do one knee-bend, count 1, 2.

R14. Side-to-side leg-stretch and bounce.

Stand with your feet apart and your hands clasped behind your buttocks. Keeping your left foot pointed forward, point your right foot to the right, turning your body until it faces right. Do 4 half knee-bends on your right leg, keeping your left leg straight. Straighten your right leg and do 4 forward bounces over your right leg, lowering your hands to the floor in front of you. Return your right foot to the original position, and point your left foot to the left. Repeat exercise to the left. Bend and straighten right leg 4 times, and bounce 4 times over straightened right leg. Repeat 4 times on left leg. Count 4 sets of 4.

R15. Feet apart—knee-bend.

Do one knee-bend, count 1, 2.

R16. Side-to-side leg-stretch and bounce.

Repeat as in R14.

R17. Feet apart—knee-bend.

Do two knee-bends, count 1, 2, 3, 4.

R18. Airplane stretch and circle.

Stand with your feet apart, fingertips touching in front of your chest, elbows out at your sides at shoulder height. Gently bring your elbows behind you as far as they can go; then return to the original position. Straighten your arms out in front of you, raise them straight up, then backwards and down, making a full circular motion. Return your arms to the original position, elbows bent and fingertips touching in front of your chest. Count to 2 as you thrust your elbows back and forth; then count 3, 4 as you circle your arms around. Do 4 stretch and circles, counting 4 sets of 4.

R19. Shoulder circle.

Stand with your feet slightly apart and arms at your sides. Tighten your abdominals and slowly push your shoulders forward; then lift your shoulders up to your ears and slowly stretch your shoulders back as far as you can. Finally, lower them to their original position. Make one shoulder rotation, count 1, 2.

R20. Arm-swing.

Stand with your feet apart and arms stretched out to the sides, level with your shoulders. Swing both arms, first to the left, and then to the right, following the movement with your nose. Keeping your hips still, swing your arms back and forth 8 times, counting 4 sets of 4.

R21. Shoulders back and forth and the shrug.

Standing with your feet together and arms at your sides, push your shoulders forward, rounding them and your back. Reverse the movement, pushing your shoulders back as far as you can; then try to raise your shoulders up to your ears. Lower your shoulders and lift your head, stretching your neck.

Pull your shoulders back and forth and up and down once, count to 4.

R22. Overhead arm-stretch (variation).

Repeat as in R10.

69

(cont'd)

Stand with your feet apart and slowly lower your arms to your sides, relaxing as the music ends.

Once-Over Lightly Routine

This is a six-minute exercise routine which will work many muscles. Lower-back muscles are not included here; lower back exercises will be added later in the program.

This routine should be done to music. We have chosen Gloria Gaynor's "Honey Bee," from her album *Never Can Say Good-Bye*. The song is exactly six minutes long, is very fast-paced, and will make the exercising much more fun.

Here are thirteen new exercises, not included in the previous pages. The remaining exercises have all been listed.

90. Run in place

Do exactly that.

91. Jump—feet apart, together

Jump twice, landing with your feet apart, then jump twice, landing with your feet together.

92. Jump—feet scissor

Jump, landing with your right foot in front of your left foot and with your weight evenly distributed on both feet. Jump again, landing with your left foot in front of your right, your weight again evenly distributed on both feet.

93. Overhead arm-bounce, circle down and around

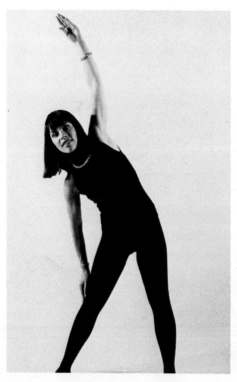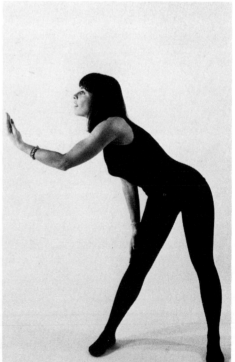

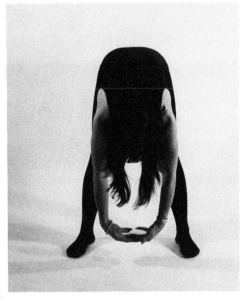
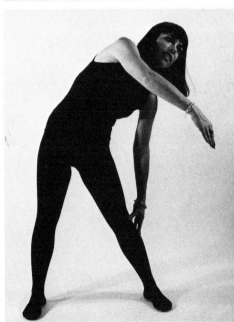
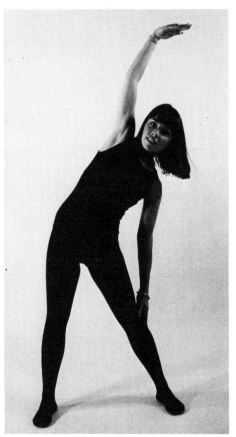

Stand with your feet apart. Keeping your right arm at your right side, raise your left arm, stretching it over your head and bounce your torso once to the right. Then twist your body so that it faces right (without moving feet or legs), and bring your left arm down and around in a full circular motion. Lower your body from the hips until you are bending forward, your hands hanging to the floor. Continue your body's circular motion to the left, raising your right arm out to the side and then up until it is above your head. Now you are in a side-bounce position, with your left arm at your side and your right arm stretched straight over your head. Bounce your torso once to the left; then reverse your position, going from left to right.

71

94. Jump—feet together

Jump up and down with your feet together.

95. Deep, deep knee-bend, crossover

Hold your arms out at a 90-degree angle from your sides; then stretch out your right leg while doing a deep knee-bend with your left leg. Being careful not to topple over, change your position, bending your right leg while stretching out your left.

96. Standing—hand walk-out and droop

The image is that of an ape walking on its hands, while its legs remain stationary. Get down on your hands and feet, your palms flat on the floor. Begin to walk forward on your palms, keeping your feet stationary; take 3 hand steps and then droop your pelvis toward the floor. (Throughout, your arms should remain straight.) Walk backwards three hand steps and stand up straight.

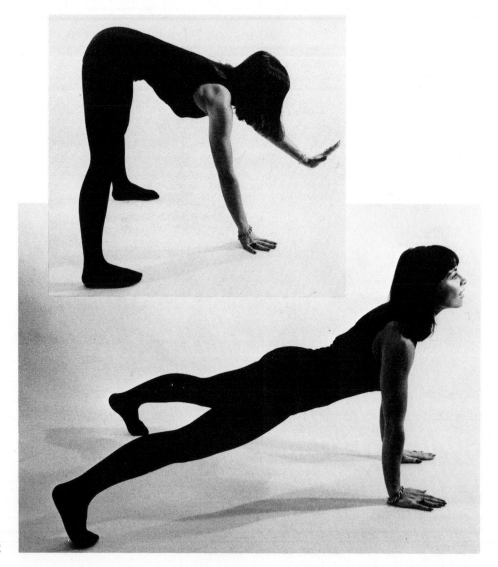

97. Standing—jump squat, jump feet apart and behind, jump squat to stand

Stand with your feet apart and jump down into a squatting position, resting your palms on the floor beside your feet. Put your weight on your hands; then kick your feet out behind you, landing with your legs straight out behind you and your feet apart. Keeping your weight on your palms, jump back into a squatting position, this time with your knees under you and your hands beside your feet. Stand up.

98. Grab-knee sit-ups

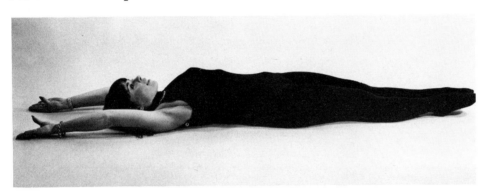

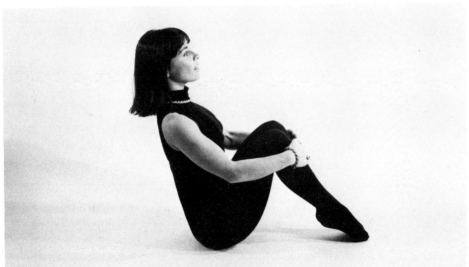

Lie supine, arms stretched out above your head and legs straight. In one motion, swing your arms up over your head and draw your knees up to your chest. Grab your knees (or shins) with your hands and tighten your abdominal muscles. Hold for a moment, and return to the original position.

99. Bent-knee crab-lift, one arm

Sit on the floor with your feet apart, legs bent, and knees up. Each leg will form a triangle with the floor. Place your right palm on the floor behind you. Bend your left arm, pressing the tricep against your chest, and raise your fist toward the ceiling. Lift your buttocks off the floor, and straighten your left arm up into the air. Return to the original sitting position.

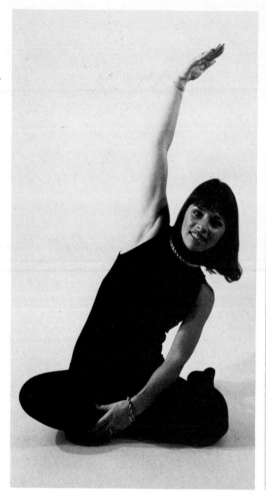
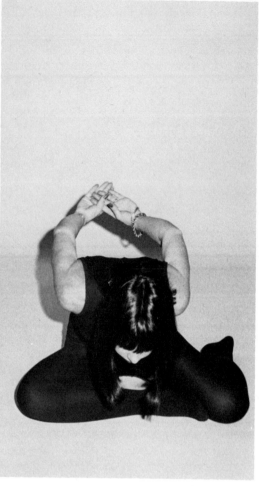

Sit with your right leg bent, the calf facing your crotch, and your left leg bent to the side. Place your right sole on your left knee and bring your left foot just past your buttocks. Raise your right arm straight up into the air, and grab your right ankle with your left hand. Bounce your torso to the left 4 times, and then bring both palms together above your head. Now lower your arms out to the sides, and then clasp your hands behind your lower back. Bounce forward twice.

101. On knees—lean back, thrust forward

Get down on your hands and knees; stretch your arms straight out in front of you as far as you can, resting your buttocks on your heels. Push your torso forward, supporting yourself on straight arms and legs bent at the knees. Return to original position.

102. Overhead arm-bounce

Stand with your feet apart and raise your left arm. Place your right hand against the right side of your right knee, and arc your left arm over your head. Bounce your torso to the right 16 times; then reverse sides.

74

1. Hip-wag (32 times)
2. Run in place (32 steps)
3. Arm-swing (16 times)
4. The swim (32 times)
5. Jump—feet apart, together (2 times)
6. Jump—feet scissors (4 times)
7. Overhead arm-bounce (8 times)
8. Overhead arm-bounce, circle down and around (4 times)
9. Run in place (16 times)
10. Jump—feet together (8 times)
11. Airplane stretch (16 times)
12. Overhead arm-bounce (8 times)
13. Overhead arm-bounce, circle down and around (4 times)
14. Side-to-side knee-bend (16 times)
15. Deep, deep knee-bend, crossover (4 times)
16. Standing—hand walk-out and droop (4 times)
17. Standing—jump squat, jump feet apart and behind, jump squat to stand (4 times)
18. Sit-ups (4 times)
19. Grab-knee sit-ups (4 times)
20. Sitting—side-to-side bounce, ear to knee (8 times)
21. Bent-knee crab-lift, one arm (4 times)
22. Sitting, L position—side and forward bounce (do series 4 times)
23. On knees—lean back, thrust forward (2 times)
24. Paint the wall (8 times)
25. Donkey-kick—knee-to-nose (8 times)
26. Head down—knee-bend (4 times)
27. Arm-swing (8 times)

Put the music on and start the routine, standing with feet apart and arms at your sides.

R1. Hip-wag.

Stand with your feet apart and arms raised slightly from your sides. Push your right hip to the right, leaning most of your weight on your straight right leg and foot. Reverse direction, doing exactly the same to the left. Get a rhythm going, wagging your hips from right to left, 32 times, counting 4 sets of 8.

R2. Run in place.

Run in place for 32 steps, counting 4 sets of 8.

R3. Arm-swing.

Stand with your feet apart and arms stretched out to the sides level with your shoulders. Swing both arms, first to the left and then to the right, following the movement with your nose. Throughout, keep your hips from moving. Swing your arms 16 times, counting (halftime) 4 sets of 4.

R4. The swim.

Stand with your feet apart, and bend forward from your hips. Move your arms in the swimming motion, with complete circular movements. Swim 8 times forward, 8 times to the right, 8 times to the left, and 8 times forward again. Count 4 sets of 8.

R5. Jump—feet apart, together.

Jump twice, landing with your feet apart, then jump twice, landing with your feet together. Do once, counting to 4.

R6. Jump—feet scissors.

Jump, landing with your right foot in front of your left foot and your weight evenly distributed on both feet. Jump again, landing with your left foot in front of the right, with your weight again evenly distributed. Do 4 times, counting to 4.

Repeat R5 and R6 twice.

R7. Overhead arm-bounce.

Stand with your feet apart and raise your left arm. Place your right hand against the right side of your right knee, and arc your left arm over your head. Bounce your torso to the right; then reverse sides. Bounce 4 times to the right and 4 times to the left, counting 2 sets of 4.

R8. Overhead arm-bounce, circle down and around
(see illustrations on pages 70–71).

Stand with your feet apart. Keeping your right arm at your right side, raise your left arm, stretching it over your head and bounce your torso once to the right. Then twist your body so that it faces right (without moving feet or legs), and bring your left arm down and around in a full circular motion. Lower your body from the hips until you are bending forward, hands hanging to the floor. Continue your body's circular motion to the left, raising your right arm out to the side and then up until it is above your head. Now you are in a side-bounce position with your left arm at your side and your right arm stretched straight over your head. Bounce your torso once to the left; then reverse your position, going from left to right.

Do four times, alternating the direction. Count 4 sets of 4.

R9. Run in place.

Run in place for 8 steps; count 8.

R10. Jump—feet together.

Jump up and down with your feet together, 4 times counting to 8 (counting to 4 halftime).

Repeat R9 and R5 twice.

R11. Airplane stretch.

Standing with your feet apart, bring your arms up to shoulder height. Bend them at the elbows until your fingers touch in front of you. Quickly bring your elbows back as far as possible, then return them to starting position. Straighten your arms out to the sides at shoulder height and turn your palms upward. Return to original position. Do 16, counting 4 sets of 4.

R12. Overhead arm-bounce.
Repeat as in R7.

R13. Overhead arm-bounce, circle down and around.
Repeat as in R8.

R14. Side-to-side knee-bend.
Stand with your feet apart and arms at your sides. Bend your left knee, leaning your weight on your left leg, keeping your right leg straight. Change sides, bending your right leg, keeping your left leg straight. Bend 4 times to the right and 4 times to the left, repeating twice. Count 4 sets of 4.

R15. Deep, deep knee-bend, crossover.
Hold your arms out at a 90-degree angle from your sides; stretch out your right leg while doing a deep knee-bend with your left. Being careful not to topple over, reverse the position. Do a deep knee-bend to the right and count 2; then swing to the left and count 2. Swing to the right again, counting 2, and to the left and stand, counting 2. Total count is 2 sets of 4.

R16. Standing—hand walk-out and droop.
Bend forward and place your right hand on the floor in front of you. Begin to walk forward on your palms, keeping your feet stationary and your legs straight. Take 3 hand steps; then droop your pelvis toward the floor. Throughout, your arms should remain straight. Walk backwards 3 hand steps and stand straight. Repeat 4 times, counting 4 sets of 8.

R17. Standing—jump squat, jump feet apart and behind,
jump squat to stand.
Stand with your feet apart and jump down into a squatting position, putting your palms on the floor beside your feet. Shift your weight to your hands; then kick your feet out behind you, landing with your legs straight out behind and your feet apart. Keeping your weight on your palms, jump back into a squatting position, your knees bent under you and your hands beside your feet. Stand up. Repeat 4 times, counting 4 sets of 4.

As you finish the last move in R17, do not stand up. Instead sit down with feet outstretched in front of you.

R18. Sit-ups.
Sit on the floor with straight legs; cross your hands over your chest and lie down. Stretch your hands above your head on the floor behind, to the count of 4. Swing your arms up above your head and sit up, keeping your legs straight and bouncing your torso forward to touch your toes with your fingers to the count of 4. Repeat 4 times, counting 4 sets of 8.

R19. Grab-knee sit-ups.
Sit on the floor with knees bent. Slowly lie down, stretching your arms above your head and straightening your legs to a count of 4. In one motion, swing your arms over your head and draw your knees up to your chest. Grab your knees (or shins) and tighten your abdominal muscles. Lie down to the count of 4 and sit up and hold your legs to the count of 4. Repeat 4 times, counting 4 sets of 8.

R20. Sitting—side-to-side bounce, ear to knee.

Sit with your legs apart and stretched out straight. Hold your right leg with both hands and, while keeping the knee straight, bounce your torso over your right leg, trying to touch your ear to your right knee. Change direction, bouncing over your left leg, trying to touch your left ear to your left knee keeping that knee straight. Do 4 bounces to the right and 4 to the left, counting 2 sets of 4.

R21. Bent-knee crab-lift, one arm.

Sit on the floor with your feet apart, legs bent, knees up, each leg forming a triangle with the floor. Place your right palm on the floor behind you. Bend your left arm, pressing the tricep against your chest, and raise your fist toward the ceiling. Lift your buttocks off the floor, and straighten your left arm up into the air. Return to the original sitting position. Do the exercise twice, raising the left arm and twice raising the right arm, counting 2 sets of 4.

R22. Sitting, L position—side and forward bounce.

Sit with your right leg bent, the calf facing your crotch, and your left leg bent to the side. Place your right sole on your left knee, and bring your left foot just past your buttocks; get into this position to the count of 4. Raise your right arm straight up and grab your right ankle with your left hand. Bounce your torso to the left 4 times. Bring palms together above your head. Lower your arms out to the sides and clasp your hands behind your lower back; bounce forward twice. Repeat the exercise twice to the right, counting 4 as you bounce, 1 as you raise your hands, and 1 as you bring them behind you. Count 2 as you bounce forward, a total of 4 sets of 4. Change directions to the count of 4, and repeat the series twice to the left.

R23. On knees—lean back, thrust forward.

Get down on your hands and knees; stretch your arms straight out in front of you as far as you can, resting your buttocks on your heels. Push your torso forward, supporting yourself on straight arms and legs bent at the knees. Return to original position. Do twice, counting 2 sets of 4.

R24. Paint the wall.

Get down on your hands and knees. As if you had a can of paint on your right side and a paintbrush and a wall to paint on your left. Reach with your left hand under your right side. Then swing your left hand back out toward the right, lifting it as high as you can. Do 4 times with your left hand and 4 times with your right, counting 4 sets of 4.

R25. Donkey-kick—knee-to-nose.

Get down on your hands and knees, keeping your arms straight. Bring your left knee up under your body, trying to touch your nose as you lower your face to meet your knee. Kick your leg out behind you, raising it as high as you can while lifting your head. Do 4 times with your left leg and 4 times with your right, counting 4 sets of 4. After finishing the donkey kick get into

78 a squatting position.

R26. Head down—knee-bend.

With your fingertips on the floor, straighten your legs so that your bottom goes up. Return to the squatting position. Repeat 4 times and count to 8, keeping your hands on the floor until the last lift. End by standing straight.

R27. Arm-swing.

Stand with your feet apart and arms stretched out to the sides level with your shoulders. Swing both arms, first to the left and then to the right, following the movement with your nose. Throughout, keep your hips from moving. Swing your arms 8 times, counting (halftime) 2 sets of 4.

End the routine on the last count of 4 by bringing both arms down to your sides.

Facial Exercises

78. Head twist

Keeping your back straight and your arms at your sides, stretch your neck without lifting your chin. Holding your shoulders in place, slowly turn your head to the right until you are looking over your right shoulder. Go only as far as is comfortable and then slowly return to the center position. Turn slowly to the left, looking over your left shoulder; return to the center and relax your back, shoulders, and neck. Straighten up again and repeat the series 8 times.

103. Scooped cheeks

Pull in your cheeks and pucker your lips. Keeping your cheeks pulled in, move your lips into a small smile, raising the muscles above your cheeks. Hold the position for 5 seconds; then relax. Repeat the exercise 6 times. This is particularly helpful in avoiding a permanent frown.

79. Head back—open and close mouth

Gently let your head fall back so that your face is turned up toward the ceiling. Don't move the rest of your body. Slowly open your mouth as wide as you can; then close it. You should feel a pulling sensation in your neck and under your chin. Repeat 8 times.

104. By your chinny chin chins

One of the first signs of a lack of physical fitness and excess weight is a double chin. Along with regular exercise and careful dieting, add the following exercise as further insurance against an unbecoming extra chin. Stick out your chin and lower jaw; your lower front teeth should protrude just beyond the upper ones. Move your jaw in a slow and gentle circular motion. Do once in a counterclockwise direction, then a clockwise direction. Do 10 to one side and 10 to the other.

105. The blowfish

This exercise is helpful to those who have a tendency toward a hollow, haggard look, from either tension or insomnia. Suck in air, filling up your mouth and stretching out your cheeks. Hold for 5 seconds, relax, and repeat 10 times.

106. The monkey

This exercise adds flexibility to otherwise monotonous facial expressions. Keep your lips together and place your tongue against the fronts of your upper teeth. Purse your lips as if for a kiss and hold for 3 seconds. Do 8 times.

Then place your tongue against the fronts of your lower teeth and smile broadly. Hold for 3 seconds and repeat 7 times.

107. Bright eyes

This exercise enhances a bright alert look. Relax your forehead and open your eyes as wide as you can. Without moving your head or furrowing your brow, look to the right, moving only your eyes. Hold the look for 2 seconds, then look to the left with your eyes only and hold for 2 seconds. Repeat 8 times and relax.

COFFEE BREAK

108. Sitting in chair—body lift

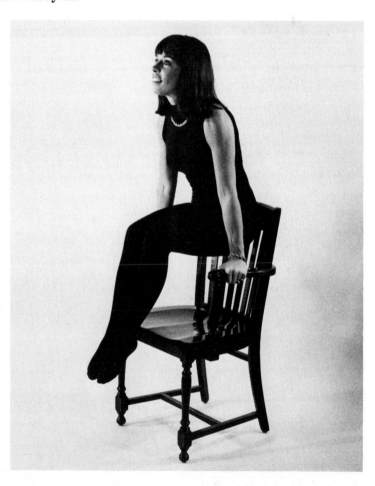

Sit down and grasp the arms of your chair with your hands. Raise your bent knees and feet off the floor and your entire torso from the seat of the chair. (Be sure that the chair arms are strong enough to support your weight.) Hold your body in the raised position for 2 seconds, then lower yourself to the seat of the chair. Repeat 4 times. As your arms and upper back become stronger, you will be able to raise your body higher. Ultimately, your arms should be absolutely straight when your body is in the raised position. This takes time, so be patient.

109. Sitting in chair—straighten legs, point and flex toes

Sit in a chair with your knees bent and your feet flat on the floor. Lift your right foot, straightening the leg out in front of you, and point your foot and toes forward. Hold for 2 seconds. Flex your foot, turning the toes upward toward the ceiling, and hold again for 2 seconds. Return your foot to the floor by bending your leg at the knee. Repeat the exercise with your left leg and foot. Then do the exercise with both legs together. Repeat 6 times.

110. Sitting in chair—forward bend, shoulder circle

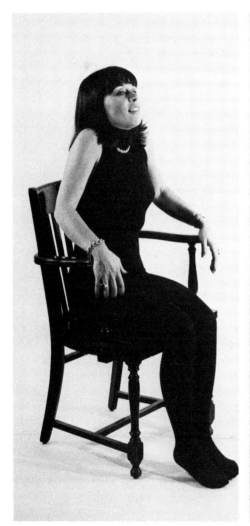 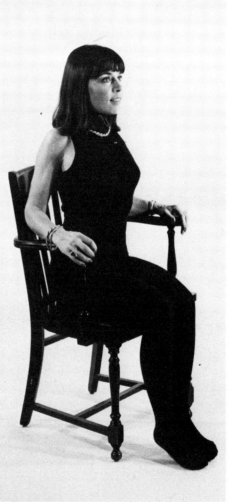

Sit in a chair with your knees bent normally. Separate the knees and rest the feet flat on the floor, about 2 feet apart. Rest your arms at your sides. As 81

(cont'd)

you bend your torso forward from the waist, round your shoulders and come as close as possible to touching your thighs. Slowly straighten your torso, at the same time moving your shoulders in a circular motion, raising them almost to your ears. Then stretch your shoulders back, and relax into your natural position. Repeat 6 times.

111. Standing, leaning on desk or chair—push-ups

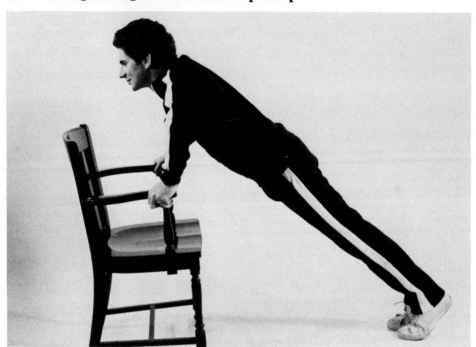

Face your desk or chair, standing at a distance of about 3 feet. With your body and your arms absolutely straight, lean forward and put your hands on the desk or on the arms of the chair. Slowly lower your chest to the desk or the chair, and then push your chest and body up to the straight-arm position. Repeat 6 times.

112. Body stretch

This can be done standing, sitting, or lying down.

A. Standing. Stretch your arms above your head, stand on your toes, and stretch your body as hard as you can. Hold the stretched position for 4 seconds and relax. Repeat 4 times.

B. Sitting. Sit with your feet flat on the floor and your knees bent. Raise your arms straight up, clasping your hands above your head, and stretch as hard as you can. Hold the stretched position for 4 seconds and relax. Repeat 4 times.

C. Lying. Lie prone or supine, your arms straight out on the floor above your head. Point your toes and stretch your body, legs, and arms as hard as you can. Hold the stretched position for 4 seconds and then relax. Repeat 4 times.

113. Sitting, straight back—knees to chest

This exercise strengthens your stomach muscles. Sit with your knees bent and feet flat on the floor. Rest your forearms on and clasp the arms of your chair with your hands. Raise your knees up toward your chest as high as you can. Hold the position for 4 seconds, and then return your feet to the floor. Repeat 4 times.

10. Head roll

Sit with your knees bent and feet flat on the floor. Rest your arms at your sides. Let your head fall forward gently without bending the upper part of your torso. Pass your right ear over your right shoulder. Then let your head fall back. Reverse and go in a counterclockwise direction. Do 5 times to the right and 5 times to the left.

114. Sitting—shoulders back and forth and shrug

Sit with your knees bent, feet flat on the floor, and arms resting at your sides. Push your shoulders forward, rounding them and your back. Reverse the movement, pushing your shoulders back as far as possible. Do 16 times. Then try to raise your shoulders up to your ears. Lower your shoulders and lift your head, stretching your neck. Do 16 times.

115. Tighten bottom and release

While sitting in a chair, tighten the gluteal muscles as hard as you can and hold them that way for 4 seconds. Repeat 6 times; try to pull in your stomach at the same time.

62. Sitting—back-push and release

Sit in a chair with your knees bent and feet flat on the floor. Rest your arms on the arms of the chair, your back supported by the back of the chair. Tighten your abdominal muscles, and slowly press the lower part of your back against the chair. Hold the position for 4 seconds, then relax stomach and back muscles. Repeat 6 to 8 times.

TRAVELING

62. Sitting—back-push and release

Sit in a chair with your knees bent and feet flat on the floor. Rest your arms on the arms of the chair, with your back supported by the back of the chair. Tighten your abdominal muscles and slowly press the lower part of your back against your chair. Hold the position for 4 seconds, then relax stomach and back muscles. Repeat 6 to 8 times.

115. Tighten bottom and release

While sitting in a chair, tighten the gluteal muscles as hard as you can, and hold them that way for 4 seconds. Repeat 6 times, trying to pull in your stomach at the same time.

116. Sitting—toe-raises

Sit in a chair with your knees bent and feet flat on the floor. (Take your shoes off for this one.) Press your heel against the floor and lift your toes, 83

(cont'd)

pulling them toward your knees. Hold the position for 4 seconds and then return your toes to the floor. Repeat 4 times. Alternate feet and repeat 4 times.

117. Sitting—heel-raises

Sit in a chair with your knees bent and feet flat on the floor. (Take your shoes off for this one, too.) Keeping your toes and the balls of your feet on the floor, raise your heel as high as you can. Hold the position for 4 seconds and release, lowering your heel to the floor. Repeat 4 times, and then alternate feet, repeating 4 times.

118. Sitting—round your shoulders

Sit in a chair with your knees bent and feet flat on the floor. Push your shoulders forward, rounding your back and tightening your pectoral muscles. Hold the position for 4 seconds, and then relax your shoulders. Repeat 4 times.

119. Sitting—shoulders back

Pull your shoulders back, stretching your chest and tightening your upper-back muscles. Hold the position for 4 seconds, and then relax your shoulders. Repeat 4 times.

120. Sitting—tighten and release chest and back

Sit in a chair with your knees bent and feet flat on the floor. Place your hands in your lap or rest your arms on the arms of your chair. Tighten and flex the muscles in your upper arms, shoulders, and upper back, and hold the position for 4 seconds. Release and relax for 2 seconds, and then repeat 6 times.

121. Sitting—one-arm tighten

Sit in a chair with your knees bent and feet flat on the floor, resting your arms on the arms of your chair. Raise your right arm, bending it at the elbow and placing your right hand behind your neck. Your elbow should be at shoulder height. Tighten and flex your upper-arm muscles and hold the position for 4 seconds. Release the muscles but keep your arm in place and repeat the exercise 4 more times. Alternate arms, and do 4 times again.

122. Sitting—tighten and release stomach

Sit in a chair with your knees bent and feet flat on the floor. Rest your hands in your lap or place your arms on the arms of your chair. Pull in and tighten your abdominal muscles; hold the position for 4 seconds and release. Repeat 6 times. Don't tighten your shoulders as you pull in your stomach.

123. Sitting—relax

Sit in a chair with your knees bent and feet flat on the floor. Rest your hands in your lap and lean back comfortably, your head against the back of your chair. Close your eyes and allow your body to relax, breathing in and out slowly and steadily. As you breath in, say, "Inhale," to yourself; as you breath out, say, "Exhale." This helps to establish a regular, relaxed rhythm. Do this for as long as you like; you may even fall asleep.

124. Lean back—leg-lift

Lean back in the tub, your back braced and your legs out straight. Hold the rim and slowly—without splashing—raise your right leg. Bend it at the knee and bring the knee as close to your chest as you can without moving your torso forward. Hold the position for 2 seconds, then return your leg to the outstretched position. Do the exercise with your left leg, and then repeat the series 6 times.

125. Feet over rim—sit-ups

Lean back in the tub, your back braced and your legs out straight, your feet on the rim of the tub in front of you. Keep your legs straight at all times. Stretch your arms straight out in front of you, and slowly move your torso forward until your hands reach your feet. Return slowly to your original position. Repeat 6 times.

126. In tub—hip-lift

Lean back in the tub, your back braced, your knees bent, and your feet flat, your legs forming triangles with the floor of the tub. Place your palms beside your buttocks, and lift your buttocks from the floor of the tub as high as you can for 4 seconds. Slowly return to your original position, and repeat the exercise 4 times.

127. Body twist

Hold your back straight and place your feet flat on the tub floor, bending your knees so that your legs form triangles with the bottom of the tub. Keeping your back straight, place your hands behind your neck. Turn your body to the right, so that you're looking over the right rim of the tub, and hold for 4 seconds. Return to your original position, and then turn your body to the left, looking over the left rim of the tub. Hold for 4 seconds, and return to the original position. Repeat 6 times.

128. Knee-bend to touch nose

Lean back in the tub, and brace your back with your legs out straight. Place your palms on the floor of the tub beside your buttocks. Bend your right leg at the knee and bring your knee up to touch your nose, leaning your torso forward to bring your nose to your knee. Hold for 2 seconds and return to your original position. Do the exercise with the left leg, and repeat the series 6 times.

OUT OF THE TUB

129. Overhead—towel bounce

Stand with your feet apart and hold a 2- to 3-foot towel at each end, pulling it taut. Raise your arms straight above your head and bounce your torso, 4 times to the right and 4 times to the left. Repeat 4 sets of bounces, keeping the towel taut and your arms straight.

130. Alternate arm-stretch

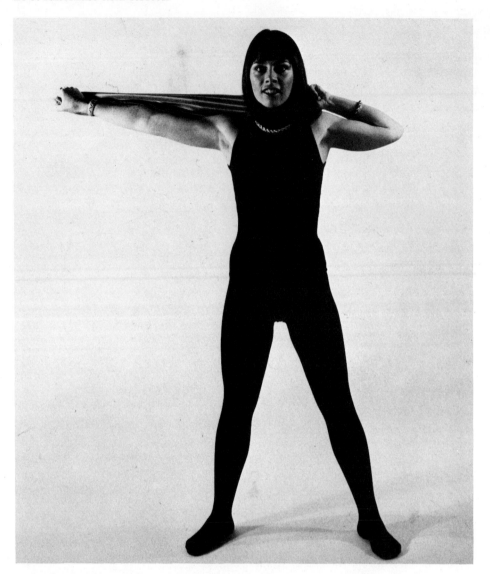

Stand with your feet apart and hold a towel taut behind you. Raise your arms to shoulder height, bending your left arm at the elbow and placing your left hand behind your head while you stretch your right arm out to the side. Keeping the towel taut, raise both arms above your head and then lower them to the left. Stretch your left arm out at shoulder height, bending your right arm at the elbow, right hand behind your head. The right elbow should be at shoulder height. Reverse the action, going from left to right. Repeat 16 times.

131. With towel—hip-wag, arm-swing

Hold a towel taut against your buttocks as you stand with feet apart and arms raised at a 45-degree angle from your thighs. Keeping your legs straight, shift your weight to your right leg, pushing your right hip to the right, and swing your arms to the left. Reverse the action, shifting your weight to your left leg, pushing your left hip to the left, and swinging your arms to the right.

The towel should be touching your buttocks at all times as if you were drying your bottom or doing the dance, "The Twist."

132. Forward kick, leg-dry

Stand with your legs straight and your feet together. As if about to dry your right leg, lean forward and place a towel on your upper thigh. Kick your straight right leg into the air in front of you and slide the towel down to your knee. Slide the towel back up to your upper thigh as you lower your foot to the floor. Repeat 4 times and alternate legs.

133. Diagonal back-dry

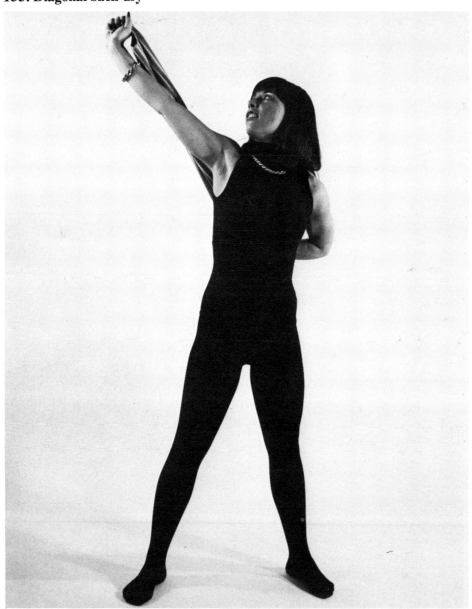

Hold a towel taut behind you, your right arm straight up in the air and your left arm, bent at the elbow, behind your back. Your left hand should be 87

(cont'd)

just between your shoulder blades. Slowly straighten your left arm, moving it down, while bending your right arm at the elbow. Your right hand should be at your right shoulder now, while your right elbow stays up in the air and your left arm is straight down, slightly behind your left side. Reverse the action, bending your left arm up and straightening your right arm. Repeat the exercise 6 times and then alternate arms. Repeat 6 times more, always keeping the towel taut.

4

Jog for Your Life and Be Fit to Sport With

In the chapter about hearts, we discussed the value of jogging as a cardiovascular exercise, but jogging is also one of the most popular outdoor activities in America.

A jog is a cross between a run and a walk, with the approximate pace and movements of a trot. The speed is somewhere between five and ten miles an hour. Jogging is neither a slimming nor a muscle-building exercise. The heart is the only muscle which jogging is meant to develop, enlarging it as well as increasing its flexibility. In order to burn up one pound of fat, one would have to expend 3,500 calories, and jogging consumes a few hundred at most. But we believe, along with many doctors, that a combined program of jogging and exercise will bring you to a peak condition of fitness.

If you absolutely hate jogging, there are many other kinds of cardiovascular activities: rope skipping and jumping, skiing, swimming, bicycling, and all-day sex. Whatever you choose is a matter of personal taste. But if you decide to jog, check first with your doctor, who can tell you what your limits are. Your heartbeat should be tested at rest and immediately after a medically directed workout.

If you shop around for medical opinions, you will undoubtedly find several contradictory ones. Probably the most well-known advocate of jogging is Dr. Kenneth Cooper of aerobics fame. Then there is Dr. Terence Kavanaugh, medical director of the Toronto Rehabilitation Centre, who has received promising results from putting heart-attack victims on a controlled program of endurance jogging.

Regardless of the skirmishes waged by wagon loads of critics against brave joggers, people all over the country continue to jog. The sale of jogging shoes, from imported Adidas to domestic Pro-Keds, has zoomed, and the "jogging look" now chic and almost de rigeur, has sparked the fashion industry. And, of course, as proof of the rage for jogging, there are the famous Boston and New York City marathons, which draw hundreds of entrants of all kinds and ages and thousands of spectators. In a recent New York City marathon, a man in his seventies and a boy of ten proudly crossed the finish line.

If you are going to integrate jogging into your daily fitness program, then you should jog at least every other day and do isotonic exercises on the days you don't jog. Jogging, like any other exercise, is progressive, and the longer you continue, the better will be the results. You should not run for either distance or speed, especially at the beginning of a jogging program.

Clothes (Help) Make the Jogger

Though we have written lightly about jogging gear, we do not disparage it. Well-fitting jogging shoes are the most important accouterments for the jogger. Make sure that the sole of the shoe you buy is made of firm rubber; it should provide support and still be flexible. The inside of the shoe should be lined with soft rubber that will cushion your foot as it absorbs the shock of impact. The heel should be neither too high nor too low. Though some joggers place their bare feet into their shoes, we recommend nice, thick, soft socks. Like soft rubber interiors, they will further cushion your feet and prevent painful blisters. When you buy jogging shoes, wear jogging socks for a good fit. Put on the shoes and jog a lap around the store. You will be testing the shoe for firmness, flexibility, and comfort. Your Achilles tendon should not be hindered by a rigid shoe, especially while jogging.

Next on the list of prerequisites for jogging are jock straps and bras. If a man prefers, he can wear snug-fitting jockey shorts instead of a jock strap. However, we have not been able to find an adequate substitute for the bra. Nothing (except perhaps a pair of hands) holds a woman in quite so well, and nothing else prevents her from bouncing painfully along. If a woman is full-breasted and jogs without a bra, she may stretch her pectoral muscles, the ones which provide essential support.

Other jogging gear is pretty much optional. Your clothing can be of any color or design that pleases you, as long as it is comfortable and loose-fitting, providing protection against the elements without creating any additional burdens. You may choose to bundle up and jog in freezing weather, but then you will be working extra hard.

You Can Do It If You Stretch

Before you put a foot outdoors, you should do special stretching exercises as preventive medicine to reduce the possibility of painfully contracted muscles. Though jogging is a superb aid to endurance activity, it lets the muscles of the legs contract, especially if one sits down after a jog. We recommend stretchercises before beginning as well as after jogging. Pre-stretching will loosen and limber legs, increase flexibility, and also prevent painful cramps. Post-stretching will similarly prevent cramps, while permitting your legs to slowly cool off; they should be sufficiently relaxed so that any subsequent activity, such as walking, will be neither painful nor difficult.

Here are our stretchercises.

The Bounce. Clasp your hands behind your back, keeping your arms straight, and bounce your trunk forward, bending at the hips. With each bounce, try to get your head closer to the ground. Do not bounce too quickly or too hard. As you reach down, nose aimed at the floor, your arms should be up behind you, aimed at the ceiling. Bounce 10 times forward, 10 times to the left, and 10 times to the right. Unclasp your hands, dangle your arms, and try to touch the floor. If you can't, do not force yourself, you will incur severe pain in the backs of your legs.

The Achilles Stretch. To stretch your Achilles tendon, as well as your calves and the fronts of your thighs, take the fencer's lunging position. The leg out in front should bend at the knee, taking the full force of the lunge. The back leg should remain straight, only leaning into the lunge. You may place your hands on your waist or simply let them dangle. Do the lunge no more than 15 times with each leg.

Rock 'n' Roll. Keeping your feet firmly on the ground and your body straight, try to move your body in a circular motion, pivoting on your ankles. Then rock from your heels to your toes, going up on your toes and back to your heels. Repeat for 10 seconds and stop.

Know How

Assuming that your doctor has given you the go-ahead to jog, you are ready to begin. Do the warm-ups from the previous chapter as well as the exercises above. At first, don't try to jog for more than ten or twelve minutes; if you have never jogged, you may wish to start by jogging fifty steps, walking fifty steps, and jogging again. Under no circumstances, even if you are impetuously optimistic, should you sprint. It may be your last. If you are completely and utterly out of shape, you need not hide in front of a television or bury your nose in a geriatric journal. Rather, you can put on your anonymous civies and go for a nice long walk to build up to jogging capacity.

Incidentally, there is no set time for walking; you may choose to do it for a week or a month, before you are ready for jogging. But if you do spend several weeks walking, then try to increase your distance gradually, day by day.

When you jog, don't carry yourself rigidly. Don't pull your shoulders up as if they are earmuffs. Don't hunch your back, unless it's Halloween and you do a great Quasimodo. And don't curl your toes under or make angry fists. Remember: Jogging is fun and it's good for you. Try not to land on your toes while jogging—toes are too delicate to absorb the full impact. Instead, as you land on your heels, try to come down as if rolling your foot from heel to toe in one graceful motion. Toes are essentially used for balance as well as like small springs, projecting you off the ground and into subsequent motion.

Since jogging is neither ballet nor running, you should not leap through the air like a gazelle. Leaps are showy, but they put an extra strain on a jogger's leg muscles. Arms are like metronomes, setting the pace for one's legs. In addition, they provide essential balance. Your arms should be pumping in time with your leg movements. If they swing wildly up and down, you will start to sprint without even realizing it. Try not to fling them from side to side. Think of yourself as one package, with all the pieces moving as a coordinated whole.

91

When jogging, breathe in through your nose; the nasal passages filter the air and adjust its temperature to that of the body. The rhythm of breathing, like the swinging of arms, should be timed to your pace. Do not huff and puff, that in itself is exhausting, and do not take long breaths and hold them until you are about to drop. If you breathe out through your mouth, you will be able to talk, mumble, or sing while you are jogging.

Do not jog immediately after eating because one's blood is concentrated in and around the digestive tract. This leaves the legs with an inadequate supply of blood. As a result, there may be pain in the leg muscles, and the stomach may become upset, perhaps leading to nausea.

If the temperature is above eighty degrees Fahrenheit, do not jog, especially if you have a heart condition. Another note of caution: Jogging uphill requires extra work, and it may be too much for some of you, at least at the beginning. Don't be embarrassed to walk up hills. And if you are in a high altitude, don't jog at all; the air is too thin and inadequate for jogging.

As you reach the concluding minutes of your jog, slow your pace and begin to shake the contractions out of your arms. When almost down to a walk, roll your head and neck. Ease into a walk now, letting your arms relax and dangle. Walk a while longer, and, once you have stopped, do the stretch-ercises above to help prevent painful contractions and stimulate the circulation of blood as well.

If you should wish to bathe after jogging, wait from ten to fifteen minutes. Give your body a chance to relax and cool off. Then use only warm water. Cold water can be a dangerous shock, and hot water will slow the pace of blood circulation, causing drowsiness.

Afterthoughts

Though we try to jog in nearly all kinds of weather, we have never challenged hurricane winds, eighty-degree–plus heat, or thin mountain air. In bad weather, we jump or skip rope; ten minutes of that is equal to thirty minutes of jogging. If you cannot jog for several days, begin your program again with care and common sense. If you have a physical injury, don't aggravate it by jogging. If, on the other hand, you have a passing emotional injury, jogging may dissipate it a little faster. Jogging is great for relieving tensions and depressions. And if you are active in sports, jogging can certainly increase your endurance.

Jog Chart

Keep an account of your jogging progress on our specially designed jogging chart. However, before you jog, check your heartbeat and mark the indicated box. Then make a note of the day you start, plus the time of day. After your first jog, mark down the distance covered, regardless of how long or short. Add the time you spent jogging a particular distance. Immediately after you have finished jogging, check your heartbeat again and mark it in the appropriate box. If you feel pain anywhere, make a note of it; be sure to readjust your evaluation the following day—the pain may diminish to minor stiffness. However, if the pain is in your chest, speak with a physician as soon as possible.

Date started

JOG CHART, 1ST 8 WEEKS

Date & time	Distance	Time	Heartbeat		Pain? Where?	Following day stiffness? Yes, no, where?
			before	after		

Monthly, starting with 3rd month

Date & time	Distance	Time	Heartbeat		Pain? Where?	Stiffness?
			before	after		

The first chart is for the first eight weeks. If possible, choose the same day each week to make your notation. The second chart is to be used on a monthly basis, beginning after the first eight weeks. Again, try to choose the same day of each month.

Your progress, if you're careful and consistent, will please you.

Be a Sport

No one makes a quick and graceful exit from a sedentary life and like magic becomes an athlete. Sports, like other physical pursuits, require a prerequisite program of daily fitness. However, sports alone will not keep you physically fit. Most sports are not performed long enough and often utilize skills of coordination rather than the whole body. But a well-exercised body has strength and endurance that can give you added power as you perform any sport. Exercise can be the difference between exhaustion after a game of tennis and energy and stamina to spare.

Tennis, in particular, requires strong flexible legs, and a healthy heart. You need a tight grip at the end of a strong arm. Well-developed pectoral muscles add power to any swing. Tennis is the fastest growing sport in the United States. One reason for its increasing popularity is its fast physical pace that provides a release in otherwise sedentary lives. The other is its keen sense of competition, a reflection of our goal-oriented society.

Tennis, however, can be dangerous for the physically unfit. The sudden, breakneck activity of a tennis game affects a sick heart the way a sudden sprint might. If you have been netted by the popularity of tennis, first get yourself into shape. Jogging, a superb endurance exercise, is a way to begin; we strongly recommend it to all athletes, whether accomplished or aspiring.

In addition to jogging, you should exercise daily and do warm-ups *before* every game. A warm muscle is twenty percent more effective than a cold muscle and can make a difference between a winning and losing game and a winning and losing body. A fitness program for tennis should include one endurance activity (jogging, swimming laps, jumping rope), a daily exercise program, and a series of pre-game warm-ups.

After a fast-paced game of tennis, put on a light sweater or jacket; quickly cooling muscles are susceptible to chills which may cause stiff muscles that lead to aches or even spasms. We suggest warm-ups after each game as well; they help keep muscles relaxed.

At the conclusion of this chapter, we have provided our special tennisises. These exercises are designed to quicken reflexes and improve motor coordination, both of which are necessary in order to play winning tennis.

The Ski Is the Limit

Skiing, by its inherent limitations, is not quite as popular as tennis, but nobody could say it is lacking in enthusiasts. From the mountains of California to those of Colorado and the Northeast, skiers take to the slopes at the drop of a chair lift.

Skiing is an exciting sport, full of speed, derring-do, and a sense of removal from everyday problems. And, as with tennis, skiing requires a body in superb physical condition. Even the best skiers have felt muscle pain, especially after the first few days on the slopes.

Since skiing utilizes muscles not fully utilized in normal activities, placing unusual stress on them, it is essential that the entire body be as finely tuned as a Stradivarius. Skiing, like tennis, is not in itself the answer to optimum fitness. You must be fit before you hit the slopes or the slopes will hit you infinitely harder. Our skiercises will increase endurance, strength, coordination, and flexibility.

There are two kinds of endurance that are absolutely necessary for the amateur skier as well as for the professional. One is cardiovascular endurance (already fully discussed); the other is the endurance of voluntary muscles which have to contract and relax repeatedly. The only way to increase this second kind of endurance is to perform specific exercises with increased repetition up to a point of proficiency beyond which exercising is superfluous. From this repetition, you will not acquire big, bulky muscles; instead, the result will be long, elegant muscles, a sure sign of flexibility and agility. We urge you to do our warm-ups, stretchercises, and flexercises.

After a day on the slopes, it is essential that you relax. Your muscles, contracting and relaxing for hours, are tired and ready to go into spasm. We recommend our series of basic warm-up exercises; they will do more for a tired body than a hot-buttered rum or a hot bath.

The Glowingness of the Cross-country Skier

Cross-country skiing—skiing on relatively level surfaces—has been increasing in popularity for the last several years. It is a superb endurance exercise, favored by those who like to avoid crowds and dangerous falls on ski slopes. And it is less expensive than regular skiing.

In many ways, cross-country skiing provides the same cardiovascular benefits as jogging. Your arms and legs are continually in motion. As the left leg shoots out, the pole in the right hand stabs the ground for balance. You alternate, right and left, as you continue moving. It sounds like a fairly simple activity but, because muscles are in constant use, it is also a tiring activity. Therefore, it is essential that you are in good condition before you try it. In fact, a few short journeys of about half an hour each, at a leisurely pace, is really the best way for the neophyte to begin. Before and after, you should do warm-ups and stretchercises. If you jog, cross-country skiing will not be as grueling as it is for those who have never undertaken any endurance sports. If you take up cross-country skiing, you'll feel wonderfully fit, and your face will glow with health and vigor.

Make a Splash

Swimming laps is one of the finest endurance exercises; it uses *all* of your voluntary muscles. It is probably the best exercise ever invented for either man or fish.

95

We have been swimming laps for years. We started with five a day, and by the end of a summer we were up to twenty-five a day. However, you must make your own judgment, for you best know your own strengths and weaknesses.

Because swimming exercises the cardiovascular system as well as the voluntary muscles, you emerge from swimming in a state of optimum fitness. Unless you have been overeating, swimming will make you look streamlined and fit. If you are overweight as well as under-exercised, don't expect to be able to swim laps without feeling tired, if not dizzy. Again, we recommend first a physical examination and then warm-ups before you take the plunge. In addition, you should do exercises which strengthen arms, shoulders, and chest. Like jogging, swimming requires patience and determination before you can expect to make progress. Swim a lap and then rest. If you reach five laps, including rests, you're on the right track to fitness and endurance.

Though one may not become another Mark Spitz, one can do as many different strokes as he did in the Olympics. You can do the crawl, backstroke, and breaststroke. If you're really a water lover, swimming below the surface offers even more variety. Once you are sufficiently strong, we recommend several laps of different strokes. This breaks the monotony and is sure to exercise all of the vital voluntary muscles. Keep in mind that speed is not your goal. Instead, pace yourself; it is *far* better to swim ten laps slowly than to race along for two laps like a motorboat. You just might run out of fuel.

My Kingdom for a Horse

Horseback riding is a splendid exercise, especially if you train yourself before you leap into the saddle. A good rider has a strong body, capable of controlling an animal weighing more than 1,000 pounds. All riders should have strong and flexible legs, arms, and hands. Flexibility and agility are extremely essential for quick movements, helping to avoid dangerous accidents. We recommend that all riders wear hard hats, especially when jumping.

Once, in the Berkshire Mountains of Massachusetts, we were cantering along on a sylvan bridle path. The day's heat was cooling into early evening, and we felt a country removed from civilization. The sound was distant, beginning almost imperceptibly like a distant thunder storm. As we rode, we heard it getting closer, its volume increasing. We assumed we were riding beside a road, and soon the rumbling sound would overtake us and pass into the distance.

Within seconds, the sound burst across us, and a motorcycle crossed not three feet in front of us. Our horses reared, panic in their eyes, and began to gallop wildly. They leapt over a nearby stream, and we could have been easily thrown. But with firm coaxing and strong control, we began to rein in the force of our animals. They slowed to a trot, then to a nervous, but exhausted walk. Their mouths foamed; their coats were lathered.

After we returned to the stables, we wiped off our own sweat and then slowly began some stretching exercises. Our muscles were not only tense from nerves, but from being in intensely contracted positions. We did exercises for our legs, backs, and arms. If we had not done those exercises, we should have had painful spasms later that night.

This does not normally happen to most people. While riding, your body moves with and against the movements of a horse, simply to avoid saddle sores; so it is important to have solid gluteal muscles. Your legs repeatedly contract to control the horse; arms and back muscles are doing the same.

A long ride requires a body in superb shape, a body that has been prepared. Riding will not, by itself, keep you fit, but it is a fine supplement to any daily fitness program.

At the end of this chapter, we have provided exercises for those of you who wish to horse around. Riding, as we have noted, requires a series of warm-ups to increase flexibility and agility. Take precautions and be in control by toning up your muscles.

We have only dealt with the most popular sports because there are too many others to include here. For all athletic endeavors there are a few basic rules to keep in mind:

1. Sports are only an integral part of any fitness program.
2. Before you take up a sport, get into optimum shape.
3. Before and after you engage in a sport, do warm-ups.
4. Endurance activities (jogging, swimming laps, jumping rope) increase your proficiency for sports.
5. While most sports are not sufficient to make you physically fit, they can add to the quality of your overall fitness.

Warning: These Sports Can be Dangerous to Your Health

Though many athletic coaches, amateur enthusiasts, and sportswriters proclaim the benefits of various sports, few of them elaborate on the dangers which can be part of any activity.

The Fate of the Careless Jogger

The careless jogger is prey to certain maladies, such as shin splints, tendonitis, and what is fast becoming known as jogger's knee.

Shin splints are due to misused muscles and sore tendons located behind the shin. This condition can be caused by wearing improper shoes which do not absorb the harsh impacts of jogging. For questions about jogging shoes, we refer you to our section on jogging clothes. Shin splints can also be caused by jogging on hard surfaces, such as cement and tar. However, if you live in a city, you may have no choice but to jog on cement and tar. If you take the time to look for alternatives, you may be fortunate enough to find a dirt track. If that is either inconvenient or nonexistent, there may be a grassy park nearby. Avoid jogging up steep hills while on hard surfaces, and if you have to jog on a hard surface, take periodic breaks.

Tendonitis is another common affliction to which joggers are especially prone. It is a familiar complaint of those who jog barefoot in the sand; your feet penetrate, rather than land, on such a surface, causing tendons to stretch. More often, tendonitis results from the Achilles tendon being jammed when the heel of the foot hits a hard surface.

Jogger's knee is an inflammation of the muscles and tendons behind the knee, often caused by neglecting warm-ups before a jog.

Jogger's knee, tendonitis, and shin splints can all result from improper shoes, jogging on hard surfaces, running on your toes, and not doing the proper warm-ups and stretchercises.

If you feel any of the above while jogging, then stop. Never continue a strenuous activity when suffering either an injury or a discomfort. Abstain from jogging for at least a week, if not longer. If you have an injury that does not heal and if you have pain, see your doctor immediately. If it is only a minor ache, let it relax. An icepack may help.

Tennis (Elbow) Anyone?

Tennis elbow has increased as a complaint as much as the popularity of the game itself. Unlike the afflictions previously mentioned, there is no sure way of avoiding it.

Doctors have failed to agree on a definition of tennis elbow, but if it is not severe and not repeatedly aggravated, it can be effectively and easily treated.

From our experience, tennis elbow seems to be caused by an inflammation in the forearm, as well as by pulled, sore muscles and tendons on the forearm side of the elbow. When the arm is continually bent at the elbow, the soreness and inflammation are aggravated. This condition seems to trouble those whose coordination is slightly off, players with a tendency to misjudge the velocity of a ball, thus swinging late. If continued, especially when backhanding, there is intense pressure on several of the muscles and tendons in the forearm.

If you think you have tennis elbow, see your doctor. Don't treat it yourself. It should be X-rayed; there may be more than only strained muscles around your elbow. Don't try to go on playing. The arm should be gently massaged and permitted to relax. Your doctor may subsequently decide to wrap it in a supportive bandage or even in a supportive splint.

Some doctors inject steroids directly into the joint of the elbow. Only you can decide what you are willing to withstand; it may be to your advantage to consult several doctors and accept something like cortisone treatment as a last resort.

Cramping Your Style

Cramps while swimming can be uncomfortable and dangerous. To avoid cramps, we suggest you take the following precautions.

Warm up before diving in for a swim so that your body will not be forced to make sudden movements. To avoid the shock of a sudden change in temperature, rub handfuls of water over the lower back, the armpits, and the base of the neck. While swimming, never exceed the limits of your strength or skill, especially in an ocean or a lake. Even in a swimming pool, don't swim so many laps that you emerge from the water dizzy and exhausted and risk a fall.

The combination of fatigue and cold can also cause cramps. If you ever experience a cramp in one of your major muscles and you are far from shore, then attempt to either tread water or float. Don't be embarrassed to call for help. If you are in shallow water, you may be able to slowly negotiate your way out of danger, or you can simply stand still until the pain has dissipated. Sometimes an agile, calm swimmer can massage a cramping area while either floating or treading water.

A final warning: Never eat just before going for a strenuous swim; otherwise, you may feel abdominal pain. It may not be a debilitating cramp, but if you continue to swim it could easily become one.

Down the Slopes and Into the Trees

There are two kinds of skiers who seem to collide with immovable objects: one is the tired skier who doesn't know when to stop; the other is the skier who looks everyplace but straight ahead.

In any sport, especially one as potentially dangerous as skiing, you should never perform when fatigued. Your coordination will be slightly off, and while skiing down a long, tortuous slope, you have to make split-second decisions. If you cannot, the chances of an accident are foolishly increased.

As a note of interest, the newer, shorter skis offer great maneuverability and can thus lead to fewer accidents; furthermore, they enable you to ski faster, so that you need quicker reflexes than ever.

WARM-UPS FOR JOGGING

32. Side-to-side knee-bend

Stand with your feet apart and your arms at your sides. Bend your left knee, leaning your weight on your left leg while keeping your right leg straight. Change sides, bending your right leg while keeping your left leg straight. Do 16 times.

36. Heel-up

Stand with your feet together and place your hands at your sides. Raise your right heel by going up on the ball and toes of your right foot leaning your weight on your left leg. Alternate from right foot to left foot, holding each position to a count of 3, and repeat alternation 16 times.

134. Snowplow

Stand with feet wide apart and turned inward, as if pigeon-toed. Tuck your pelvis under and forward while you bend your knees, and hold your arms up like the wings of a bird. Tilt your torso and thighs to the right, leaning

99

(cont'd)

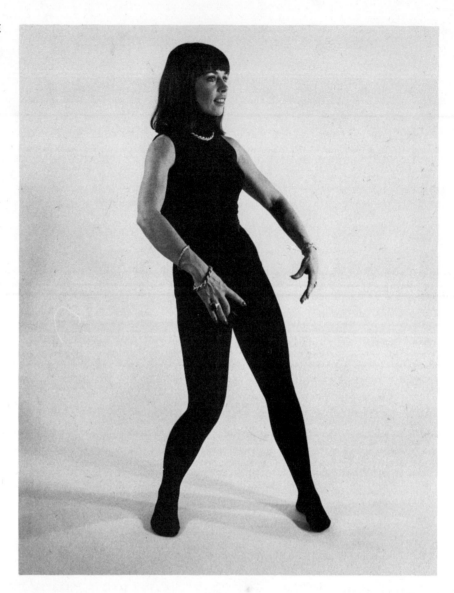

slightly backward. Your weight will be mostly on your right leg. Reverse direction, going to the left. Do each side 8 times, 16 altogether.

89. Arm-swing

Stand with your feet apart and your arms stretched out to the sides, level with your shoulders. Swing both arms, first to the left, then to the right, following this movement with your nose. Throughout, keep your hips from moving. Do 16 times.

135. Washing machine

Start with your feet apart and bend forward from the hips. Your body should make a right angle. Bend your arms at the elbows, so that they form right angles too. Twist your body up and down from the waist, moving your torso and arms like the agitating motion of a washing machine. Repeat 16 times. (See illustration on opposite page.)

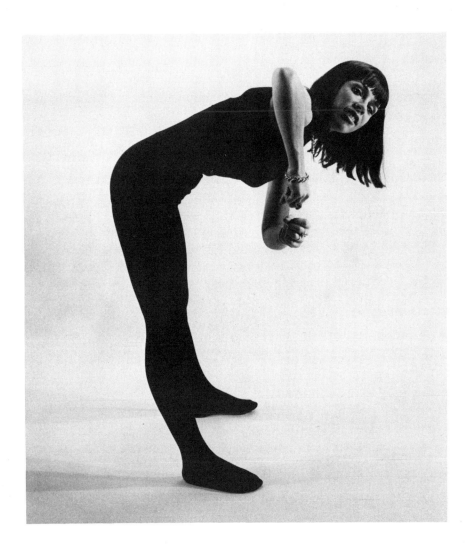

136. The touch-toe twist

Stand with your feet apart, and bend forward from the hips. Keeping your legs straight, touch the fingers of your left hand to the toes of your right foot. Your right arm should be straight up in the air. Reverse your arms and twist and touch 16 times.

25. Standing—pelvic tilt

Place your feet apart and bend your knees slightly. Place your hands on either your thighs or hips. Without moving your shoulders, push out your bottom, and then draw it under and tighten your abdominals. Do this 8 to 16 times, careful not to move your legs or shoulders.

8. Standing—forward bounce

Stand with your feet apart, legs straight, and hands clasped behind you. Bounce forward, bending at the hips, as low as you can without bending your knees. Keeping your arms straight, bring your hands up behind you as you bounce forward. Bounce 8 times forward, 8 times over the right leg, 8 times forward, 8 times over the left leg, and, finally, 8 times forward again.

101

12. The swim

Stand with your feet apart and bend forward from your hips. Move your arms in a swimming motion, making complete circular movements. Each arm should circle 16 times.

87. Overhead arm-stretch

Stand with your feet together and stretch your arms up straight above your head. Bend your right leg at the knee and stretch your right arm higher above your head, as hard and as far as you can. Hold for 4 seconds. Release your right arm, still holding it above your head, and straighten your right leg. Bend your left leg at the knee, and stretch your left arm higher above your head, as hard and as far as you can. Hold for 4 seconds. Release your left arm, still holding it above your head, and straighten your left leg. Repeat series 8 times.

102. Overhead arm-bounce

Stand with your feet apart and raise your left arm. Place your right hand against the right side of your right knee, and arc your left arm over your head. Bounce your torso to the right 16 times, then reverse sides.

88. Side-to-side leg-stretch and bounce

Stand with your feet apart and your hands clasped behind your buttocks. Keeping your left foot pointed forward, turn your right foot out to point right, and turn your body until it faces right. Do 4 half knee-bends on your right leg, keeping your left leg straight. Straighten your right leg and do 4 forward bounces over your right leg, raising your clasped hands up behind you as high as you can. Repeat series 4 times. Return your right foot to the original position, pointed forward, and turn your left foot to the left. Repeat exercise 4 times to the left.

9. Sitting—forward bounce, legs straight, feet together

Sit on the floor with your legs straight out in front of you and your feet together. Hold your legs and pull your torso forward, then release it backward. You should feel a stretching in the backs of your legs. Bounce forward and back 16 times with your toes pointed, then flex your feet so that your toes point toward the ceiling and bounce 16 times.

22. Bent-knee sit-ups

Sit on the floor with your knees bent and anchor your feet under a couch, dresser, or piece of sturdy furniture. Clasp your hands behind your neck. From the sitting position, slowly lie down. When your back is flat on the floor, sit up, keeping your hands clasped behind your neck. Be sure to come up with a rounded back; straighten your back when you have reached the final sitting position. Start with 5 and work up to a comfortable number.

137. Rope jump—feet together, double jump

Jump rope. Start by resting your rope behind your feet with your arms hanging down at your sides. Swing your rope from behind your feet up over your head and down in front of you. As the rope hits the floor in front of you, jump over it with feet together. Continue swinging the rope up behind you and jump a second time as the rope swings overhead. Jump again when the rope hits the floor. Continue jumping 2 times for every swing. Swing 20 times.

138. Rope jump—skip

Swing your rope from behind your feet up over your head and down in front of you. As the rope hits the floor in front of you, leap over it, leading with your right foot. Land on your right foot, bringing your left foot down next to it as you swing the rope up and over your head again. Step on your left foot as the rope swings forward and leap with your right foot as the rope hits the floor in front of you. Repeat 10 times with right foot and 10 times with left foot.

46A. Rope jump—feet together, single jump

Jump once for every time you swing the rope from behind your feet, over your head, and down to the floor in front of you. Repeat 12 times.

139. Rope jump—backwards

Place your rope in front of you. Swing it forward, up over your head, and back down behind your feet. As the rope hits the floor behind your feet, jump over it, pulling the rope forward, up and around again. As the rope swings over your head, jump a second time. Repeat backward jumps 20 times.

140. Rope swing—leap, hop

Swing your rope from behind your feet, up over your head and down in front of you. As the rope hits the floor, leap over it with your right foot. Land on your right foot, bringing your left foot down next to it. As you swing your rope over your head, make a small jump with feet together, and then leap over the rope with your right foot as the rope hits the floor in front of you. Leap and jump 10 times with your right foot and 10 times with your left foot.

INSTEAD OF JOGGING

141. Run in place—high knee-lift

Run in place, raising each knee as high as you can. Run 50 steps.

142. Run in place—straight leg forward

Run in place, tipping slightly backward and keeping your lifted leg as straight as possible out in front of you. This resembles the running of an ostrich. Run 50 steps.

143. Run in place—straight leg back

Run in place, leaning slightly forward as you keep the lifted leg as straight as possible while raising it behind you. This one resembles an ice skater, holding one leg perpendicular to the body and pointing backwards. Run 50 steps.

103

144. Run in place—legs to the side

Run in place, kicking each straight leg out to each side. This one resembles the pendulum of a clock. Run 50 steps.

145. Jump, squat, double upright jump

Jump down to a squatting position, resting your palms on the floor beside your feet. Leap up, then jump twice with your legs straight. Repeat series 4 times.

WARM-UPS FOR TENNIS

12. The swim

Stand with your feet apart and bend forward from your hips. Move your arms in the swimming motion, careful to make complete circular movements. Each arm should circle 16 times.

95. Deep, deep knee-bend, crossover

Hold your arms out at a 90-degree angle from your sides, then stretch out your right leg while doing a deep knee-bend with your left. Being careful not to topple over, move to your right, bending your right leg while stretching out your left. Repeat 4 times.

102. Overhead arm-bounce

Stand with your feet apart and raise your left arm. Place your right hand against the right side of your right knee, and arc your left arm over your head. Bounce your torso to the right 16 times, then reverse sides.

88. Side-to-side leg-stretch and bounce

Stand with your feet apart and your hands clasped behind your buttocks. Keeping your left foot pointed forward, turn your right foot out to point right and turn your body until it faces right. Do 4 half knee-bends on your right leg, keeping your left leg straight. Straighten your right leg and do 4 forward bounces over your right leg, raising your clasped hands up behind you as high as you can. Repeat series 4 times. Return your right foot to the original position, pointed forward, and turn your left foot to the left. Repeat exercise 4 times to the left.

22. Bent-knee sit-ups

Sit on the floor with your knees bent and anchor your feet under a couch, dresser, or piece of sturdy furniture. Clasp your hands behind your neck. From the sitting position, slowly lie down. When your back is flat on the floor, sit up, keeping your hands clasped behind your neck. Come up with a round, not a straight back, only straighten your back when you have reached the final sitting position. Start with 5 and work up to whatever is comfortable.

146. On elbow—bicycle

Lie on your right side, keeping your torso off the floor. Lean on the right side of your bottom, as well as on your right elbow and forearm. For extra balance, place the palm of your left hand on the floor behind you. Move your legs in a gentle, circular motion as if riding a bicycle. Do 16 times and
alternate sides.

147. Sitting—forward bounce, feet together, knees apart

Sit on the floor, bend your legs, and put the soles of your feet together. Grasp your ankles, keep your back straight, and rock your torso back and forth. Repeat 6 times. Then round your back and shoulders, pull your forehead toward your toes, and bounce an additional 6 times.

68. Dowel—arm-swing

Stand with your feet apart, holding the 3-foot dowel at each end in front of your chest. The dowel should be horizontal with the floor. Keeping your arms at shoulder height, swing from side to side, following the motion of your arms with your head. Keep your hips and thighs stationary, and do 16 times.

148. Dowel—overhead arm-bounce

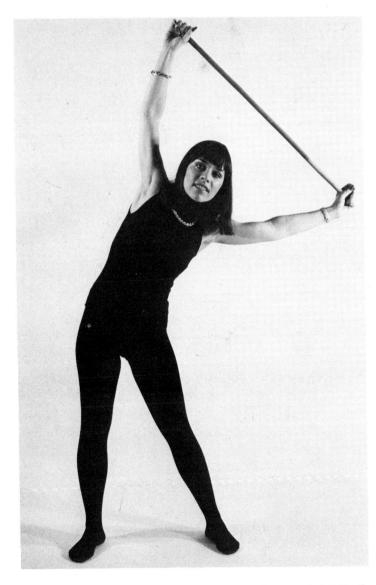

Stand with your feet apart. Grasping the dowel at each end, hold it directly above your head with your arms absolutely straight. Keeping your legs 105

(cont'd)

straight, lean your torso from side to side, creating an arc motion with the dowel. Go from side to side 4 times, then bounce 4 times to the right and 4 times to the left.

75. Dowel—shoulder rotate

Keeping your arms straight, hold a 3-foot dowel at each end in front of your thighs. Slowly raise your arms up in front of you and then straight up over your head. Slowly continue moving your arms back as far as you can, always keeping those arms straight. Never force your arms back or up in the straight position. Be sure to go only as far as you can comfortably. If you feel pain you've gone too far and should bend your arms and lower them until the dowel is just behind your buttocks and your arms are straight again. Slowly raise your straight arms up behind you as far as you can. When your arms cannot go any further up without pain, bend them at the elbows and continue raising them until they stretch straight up over your head. Slowly lower your straight arms in front of you until the dowel is against your upper thighs. Do 16 times. After several weeks, you should be able to do this exercise without bending your elbows.

149. Dowel, standing—forward bounce

Stand with your feet apart. Hold the dowel at each end, but behind you this time. Make sure that your arms are straight, if not rigid. Bounce forward from your hips, lifting your arms up behind your back as far as they will go. Bounce forward 8 times, to your right 8 times, to your left 8 times. Return to a forward bounce for an additional 8 times.

WARM-UPS FOR SKIING (DOWNHILL AND CROSS-COUNTRY)

39. Curl feet and flatten

Stand with your feet together and your arms at your sides. Shift your weight to the outsides of your feet and curl your toes under. Hold for 4 seconds, then return to a flat-footed stance. Do 8 times.

31. Half knee-bend, heel-down

Stand with your feet together and your arms stretched out in front of you. Bend your knees as if doing a deep knee-bend, but only go half way down. Your heels, along with the rest of your feet, should remain flat on the floor. Do 16 times.

32. Side-to-side knee-bend

Stand with your feet apart and your arms at your sides. Bend your left knee, leaning your weight on your left leg, keeping your right leg straight. Change sides, bending your right leg, keeping your left leg straight. Do 16 times.

43. Knee-wag

Stand with your feet and knees together; bend your knees slightly and lean on the outer part of your right foot and the inner part of your left, and sway your knees to the right. Alternate the direction of your sways, moving back and forth 16 times.

25. Standing—pelvic tilt

Place feet apart and bend your knees slightly. Place your hands either on your thighs or on your hips. Without moving your shoulders, push your bottom out, then draw it under and tighten your abdominals. Do this 8 to 16 times.

134. Snowplow

Stand with your feet wide apart and turned inward, as if you are pigeon-toed. Tuck your pelvis under and forward while bending your knees. Hold your arms up like the wings of a bird. Tilt your torso and thighs to the right, leaning slightly backward, your weight mostly on your right leg. Then reverse direction. Do each side 8 times, or 16 altogether.

44. Snowplow, knee-bend

Stand with your feet apart and turned inward as if you are pigeon-toed. Your knees and thighs should be touching and your calves should be apart. Stand up, straightening your legs. Do 16 times.

150. Standing—ostrich kick

Stand with your feet apart and your arms straight out in front of you at shoulder height. Bend your right leg slightly at the knee, and kick your straight left leg so that the toes touch your right palm or fingers. Place your left foot on the floor again and bend the left leg slightly at the knee. Kick your straight right leg so that the toes touch your left palm or fingers. Place your right foot on the floor, and repeat series 8 times.

8. Standing—forward bounce

Stand with your feet apart, legs straight, and hands clasped behind you. Bounce forward, bending at the hips, as low as you comfortably can without bending your knees. Keeping your arms straight, bring your hands up behind you as you bounce forward. Bounce 8 times forward, 8 times over the right leg, 8 times forward, 8 times over the left leg, and, finally 8 times forward again.

19. Airplane stretch

Standing with your feet apart, bring your arms up to shoulder height and bend them at the elbows until your fingers touch in front of you. Quickly bring your elbows back as far as you can, and then return them to starting position with your hands in front of you. Straighten your arms out to the sides, keeping them at shoulder height, and turn your palms upward. Return to original position and repeat 12 times.

135. Washing machine

Start with your feet apart, and bend forward from the hips, your body making a right angle. Bend your arms at the elbows so that they form right angles, too. Twist your body up and down from the waist, moving your torso and arms like the agitating motion of a washing machine. Repeat 16 times.

22. Bent-knee sit-ups

Sit on the floor with your knees bent, and anchor your feet under a couch, dresser, or piece of sturdy furniture. Clasp your hands behind your neck. From a sitting position, slowly lie down. When your back is flat on the floor, sit up, keeping your hands clasped behind your neck. Come up with a round back, straightening your back when you have reached the final sitting position. Start with 5 and work up to whatever is comfortable.

24. On elbows—knees to chest, straighten, and circle

Sit on the floor, and then lean back on your elbows and forearms. Bend your knees over your chest. Release, straightening your legs upward, and then slowly separate them. As they separate and lower, they will form a circle in the air. Bring the legs together about 4 to 6 inches from the floor and hold for 3 seconds. Repeat the exercise 4 times. Each week, add an additonal rotation, but if you feel lower-back pain at any time, *stop*. Do this exercise a few weeks into the program, when your muscles are stronger and your body is in better shape.

6. Prone—leg-lifts

Lie prone, resting your chin on folded arms. Keeping your hipbones on the floor, raise your right leg without bending the knee. Hold your leg in the air for 2 seconds; then lower it. Raise your left leg in the same manner. Repeat 16 times.

4. Prone—arm-lifts

Lie prone with your chin on the floor and your arms stretched out in front of you. Lift your right arm into the air as high as you can, keeping it beside your ear and keeping your chin on the floor. Lower your right arm; then lift the left arm in the same manner. Repeat 16 times.

1. Back flat—leg-lower

Lie supine. Bring your knees over your chest, and then straighten your legs so that they form a 90-degree angle with your torso and the floor. Keeping the small of your back pressed firmly against the floor, slowly lower your legs *only* as far as you can without your back rising off the floor. (If you feel your back rising, you have lowered your legs too far.) When you reach that point, hold for 4 seconds; then release by bending your knees over your chest. Rest and repeat 4 times. *Never* lower your legs all the way down to the floor, for that will cause back strain. Be sure you go only as far as you can while keeping your back flat.

For illustration see page 15.

WARM-UPS FOR SWIMMING: OUT OF THE WATER

12. The swim

Stand with your feet apart and bend forward from the hips. Move your arms in the swimming motion, making complete circular movements. Each arm should circle 16 times.

19. Airplane stretch

Standing with your feet apart, bring your arms up to shoulder height, bending them at the elbows until your fingers touch in front of you. Quickly, bring your elbows back as far as you can, then return them to the starting position with your hands in front of you. Straighten your arms out to the sides, keeping them at shoulder height, and turn your palms upward. Return to original position and repeat 12 times.

136. The touch-toe twist

Stand with your feet apart and bend forward from the hips, keeping your legs straight. Touch the fingers of your left hand to the toes of your right foot, with your right arm sticking straight up into the air. Reverse your arms, and twist and touch 16 times.

89. Arm-swing

Stand with your feet apart and your arms stretched out to the sides, level with your shoulders. Swing both arms, first to the left and then to the right, following the movement with your nose. Throughout, keep your hips from moving. Do 16 times.

18. The back of my hand

This exercise can be done with feet together or apart. Keep your left arm at your side and raise your right arm, bending it at the elbow. Place the back of your right hand against your right cheek. Swing your arm, throwing your hand back and away from your face until your arm is as straight as a back-stroker's. Do the same with your left hand and arm, leaving your right at your side. Do 8 times with each arm.

151. Prone—alternate leg-and-arm–lift

Lie prone, your chin on the floor, and stretch your arms straight out in front of you. Lift your straight left arm and your straight right leg simultaneously. As your arm rises, it should remain beside your head; as your leg rises, your hipbone should stay on the floor. Hold for 2 seconds, then lower your arm and leg and reverse sides, lifting your straight right arm and straight left leg. Do 8 times.

47. On elbows—frog kick

Sit on the floor and lean back on your elbows and forearms. Bend your legs at the knees and bring your knees over your chest. Slowly separate your knees and place the soles of your feet together. Separate your legs and feet, straightening out your legs like open scissors blades. Close those scissors, bringing your legs and feet together again about 6 to 8 inches from the floor. Hold for 2 seconds. Return to the second position, with your legs bent over your chest. Do 8 times; stop if you feel any strain or pain in your lower back.

48. On elbows—scissors crossover

Sit on the floor and lean back on your elbows and forearms. With legs apart, raise them off the floor and flex your feet, turning your toes outward. Then turn your toes inward to face each other and cross your left leg over your right. From the completed crossover position, turn your feet outward 109

(cont'd)

and move your legs apart again. Keeping your straight legs off the floor, reverse the order, passing your right foot over your left. Do 8 times. Stop if you feel any lower-back pain.

102. Overhead arm-bounce

Stand with your feet apart and raise your left arm. Place your right hand against the right side of your knee, and arc your left arm over your head. Bounce your torso to the right 16 times; then reverse sides.

WARM-UPS FOR SWIMMING: IN THE WATER

152. Legs raised, knees bent, and straighten

Stand against the pool wall in shoulder-height water. Hold the edge of the pool behind you and slowly raise your knees to your chest. Straighten your legs out in front of you, then slowly return them to a standing position, feet touching the bottom of the pool. Repeat 8 times.

153. Side-to-side leg-lifts

Stand in chest-level water and face one wall of the pool. Place your hands on the edge of the pool and lean your weight on your left foot, raising your straight right leg out and up to the side as high as you can. Point your foot and then slowly lower your straight leg. Repeat 6 times, then change legs.

154. Frog kick

Stand in chest-level water with your back against one wall of the pool. Holding the edge of the pool behind you, slowly raise your legs straight up in front of you until they are perpendicular to your body. Slowly separate your legs and bend your knees, drawing your feet up toward your crotch. When you cannot bend your knees further, slowly swing your feet out to the sides, straightening your legs. Bring your straight legs together, again perpendicular to your body. Repeat 6 times.

155. Standing scissors

Stand in shoulder-height water, facing one wall of the pool, and place your hands on the edge of the pool. Lift your feet off the pool floor resting your weight on bent arms and, with toes pointed, slowly open and close your straight legs like a pair of scissors. Repeat 12 times.

156. Scissor foot-slide against pool wall

This exercise can only be done if the pool wall is either tile or vinyl. Cement may scrape the skin on your feet. Stand in chest-level water facing the wall of the pool and place your hands on the pool's edge. With straight legs, place your feet on the wall in front of you and push your buttocks out into the water without submerging your head and without letting go of the pool's edge. Slowly spread your straight legs as wide as you can, then slowly bring your feet and legs together again. Repeat 6 times.

157. Floating scissor kick

Stand in chest-level water, facing the wall of the pool, and place your hands on the edge of the pool. Slowly raise your body and legs out behind you, away from the pool wall, until you are floating. Holding the edge of the pool, do the scissor kick, keeping your legs straight. Do 24 times.

158. Floating side-scissor kick

Stand in chest-level water, facing the wall of the pool, and place your hands on the edge of the pool. Slowly raise your body and legs away from the wall, turning until you are floating on your right side. Holding the pool's edge, do the scissor kick, moving your straight legs back and forth so that they pass each other 24 times. Turn over to float on your left side, and repeat the scissor kick 24 times.

159. Bent-knee rudder

Stand in chest-level water, facing the wall of the pool, and place your hands on the edge of the pool. Lean your weight on your left leg, bending your right leg at the knee; place your right foot on the inside of your left knee. As if your bent right leg were the rudder of a boat, slowly shift it back and forth. Do this rudder swing 12 times, and then alternate legs. Do 12 rudder swings with your left leg.

160. Straight-leg circle

Stand in chest-level water, facing the wall of the pool at a distance of a foot, and hold the edge of the pool with both hands. Lean your weight on your left leg and raise your right leg from the pool floor, slightly to your right. Make small circular motions with your straight right leg, clockwise 10 times and counterclockwise 10 times. Return your right foot to the floor, lean your weight on it, and raise your left foot, making the same circular motions with your straight left leg. Do 10 clockwise and 10 counterclockwise circles.

WARM-UPS FOR RIDING

161. Sitting on chair—tighten and release

Straddle a straight-backed chair, one without arms, facing its back and grasping the top of it. Press your legs against the sides of the chair, tightening all the muscles along your inner thigh. Hold for 6 seconds, then relax. Repeat 6 times.

162. On knees—pelvic tilt

Kneel down resting your weight on your knees, shins, and insteps, keeping your legs slightly apart. Without moving your shoulders, push out your bottom and then tuck it under, contracting your stomach muscles. Do 12 times.

163. Sit-ups holding ball between knees

Sit on the floor with your knees bent, and anchor your feet under a couch, dresser, or any piece of sturdy furniture. Place a ball—about 10 to 12 inches in diameter—between your knees. Holding the ball between your knees, clasp your hands behind your neck, and from a sitting position slowly lie down. When your back is flat on the floor, sit up, keeping your hands behind your neck and the ball tightly between your knees. Come up with a rounded back,

111

(cont'd)

straightening your back when you have reached the final sitting position. Start with 5 sit-ups and work up to whatever is comfortable.

164. On elbows—leg-lifts with ball between ankles

Sit on the floor and place a ball—about 10 to 12 inches in diameter—between your ankles. Lean back on your elbows, and, with the ball tightly between your ankles, bend your knees up to your chest. Then straighten your legs out in front of you, your feet about 2 feet off the floor. Hold your legs straight for 4 seconds; then bend your knees again. Repeat 6 times.

165. On elbows—side-to-side body shift with ball between ankles

Sit on the floor and place a ball—about 10 to 12 inches in diameter—between your ankles. Lean back on your elbows and raise your straight legs up about 2 feet from the floor. Keeping your legs in the air and the ball between your ankles, roll over onto your right side, leaning on your right buttock, right elbow, and right forearm with your left hand behind you for balance. Your legs should still be in the air, the right one about 1 foot from the floor and the left one about 2 feet from the floor. Hold yourself on your right side for 2 seconds, then roll over onto your left, leaning on your left buttock, elbow, and forearm with your right hand behind you for balance. Your left foot should be about 1 foot from the floor and your right 2 feet from the floor. Hold the position on your left side for 2 seconds; then return to your right side. Repeat 8 times.

147. Sitting—forward bounce, feet together, knees apart

Sit on the floor, bend your legs, and put the soles of your feet together. Grasp your ankles, keeping your back straight, and rock your torso back and forth. Repeat motion 6 times. Then round your back and shoulders, pull your forehead toward your toes, and bounce another 6 times.

35. On side—under leg-lift

Lie on your right side with your head on your right bicep to cushion your head from the floor. Bend your left leg, placing your left foot behind your right knee. Lift your right leg as far as you can and lower it. Do 6 times with toes pointed, and 6 times with foot flexed. Change sides and repeat, raising the left foot and bending the right leg.

60. Elbow snap

Stand with your legs apart, your arms at shoulder height and bent at the elbows. Twist your torso twice to the right and twice to the left, keeping your legs and hips stationary. Twist 16 times in each direction.

135. Washing machine

Start with your feet apart, and bend forward from the hips, your body making a right angle. Bend your arms at the elbows, so that they form right angles, too. Twist your body up and down from the waist, moving your torso and arms like the agitating motion of a washing machine. Repeat 16 times.

16. Let-downs

Get into the push-up position, body straight out, supported on straight
arms and toes. Slowly bend your arms and lower your body to the floor,

keeping yourself straight while you count to 6. When you reach the floor, relax for a few seconds; then return to your starting position, but not by doing a push-up. Repeat the let-down 4 to 6 times.

27. Back—arch and flatten

Lie supine. Bend your knees to a 90-degree angle, and keep your feet flat on the floor. With your upper back and bottom on the floor, gently arch your lower back. Then flatten it, gently pressing it against the floor. Hold the flattened position for 4 seconds, and repeat the entire exercise 6 times.

5

The Joy of Sexercising

Though the word, sexercise, may have a mechanical connotation, vis-à-vis the spontaneity of sexual intercourse, our purpose is not to decrease spontaneity but to increase ability to enjoy the results of that spontaneity. Our sexercises will enhance sexual skills and increase sexual longevity.

For men and women, satisfying sexual activity requires bodies that are agile, strong, and flexible. Sustained sexual activity requires as much endurance as many sports. We advocate jogging for improved sex, but if you prefer, jump rope, bicycle, or swim laps.

One of the surest signs of an inadequate lover is excess fat, particularly around the abdomen and buttocks. An over-padded belly is an obvious disadvantage in sexual intercourse, reducing pleasure by preventing certain areas from being touched. Furthermore, fat people have extra baggage to carry; therefore, they have less strength and endurance than lean, fit people. And since an overweight person is more likely to have arteriosclerosis, prolonged sexual intercourse may even prove dangerous.

So make sure that you and yours are trim and healthy; discourage excess fat and do an endurance activity as well as our sexercises. Remember, there is nothing that reduces sexual desire as effectively as an unattractive body.

Alcoholism is another obstacle to successful sexual activity. The inebriated man is often unable to consummate the sexual act, while the inebriated woman may be numb to the pleasures of sex.

In addition to endurance and basic attractiveness, our sexercises develop certain requisite skills such as the ability to flexibly tilt and untilt the pelvis, for which a strong stomach as well as a strong lower back are needed. The gluteal sexercises are particularly important for women, because they also exercise the vaginal muscles, enhancing their tone and flexibility. A woman with good vaginal muscles will experience pleasure she can control and also provide more pleasure to her partner.

A woman who exercises her buttocks daily will have a pleasing shape and strong groin muscles. Men should also do our isometric gluteals—a simple tightening and releasing of the gluteal muscles than can be done when traveling or sitting at a desk—for the reward is a strong, muscular buttocks.

At the end of this chapter you will find all the sexercises you will ever need, designed for your happiness by making and keeping you physically fit. Though we have left sexual technique to your own imagination, we have given you the blueprint for performing sex with endurance, flexibility, agility, and strength.

SEXERCISES

166. Togetherness—push and pull

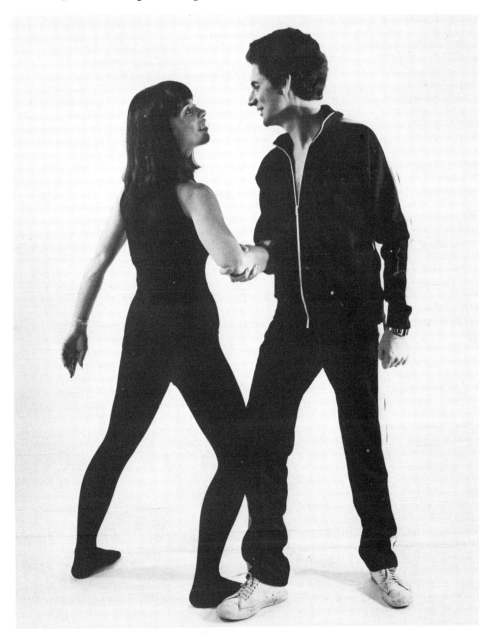

Stand next to your partner, your right sides next to each other, one facing forward while the other faces backward. Both of you stand with your feet apart, the outsides of your right feet and knees against each other's. Each

(cont'd)

keep your left arm at your side, and clasp the other's right forearm. Press your right shoulders together and gently push against each other for 4 seconds. Lean away, each putting your weight on your left leg, still grasping forearms, and pull outward for 4 seconds. Repeat 4 times, then change sides, with left sides adjoining now, and repeat 4 times.

167. Togetherness—half knee-bend

Stand facing your partner so that your toes touch and grasp each other's forearms. Lean slightly backward and bend so that your knees touch; hold that position for 2 seconds. Stand straight and repeat 6 times.

168. Togetherness—facing deep knee-bend

Stand facing your partner at a distance of about 2 feet. Clasp each other's forearms and lean slightly backward. Do a deep knee-bend, letting your heels come off the floor, and use each other's weight for balance. Return to a standing position, and repeat 4 times.

169. Togetherness—back-to-back deep knee-bend

Stand back-to-back with your heels about 4 inches away from your partner's. Link arms at the elbows, and lean back on each other's backs. Slowly do deep bends, letting your heels rise off the floor. Stand straight and repeat 4 times.

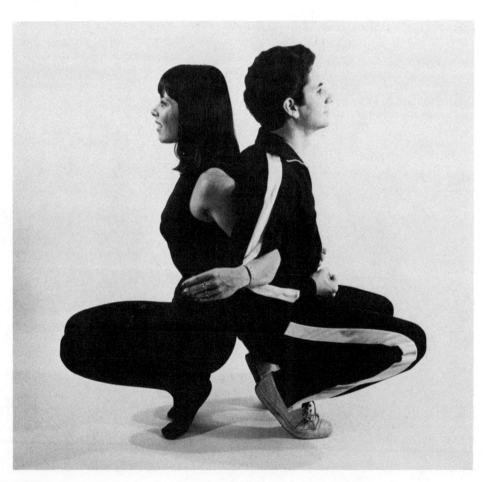

170. Row your boat

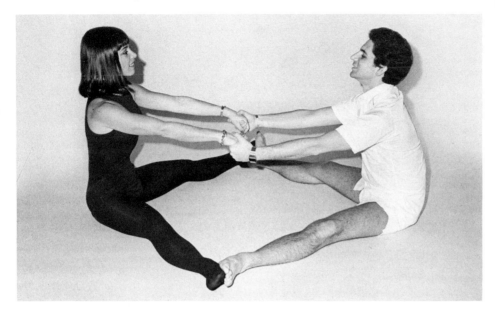

Sit on the floor and face your partner. Both spread your legs, and place your feet against each other's. Hold your partner's hands and rock forward and backward, both of you keeping your legs straight. Pull your partner forward as far as is comfortable, then let your partner pull you forward and back, both of you keeping your legs straight. You should feel muscles pull in the backs of your legs, but not pain. Repeat rocking motion 16 times.

171. Row your boat with bent knees

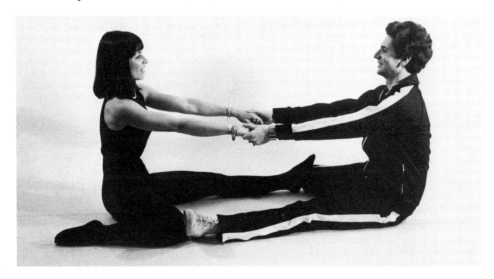

Sit on the floor and face your partner. Bend your right leg, placing your right foot beside the right side of your buttocks. Place your partner's left foot on your right knee. Your partner should also bend the right leg, placing the right foot beside the buttocks. Place your left foot on your partner's right knee, and rock back and forth 16 times; then reverse legs.

117

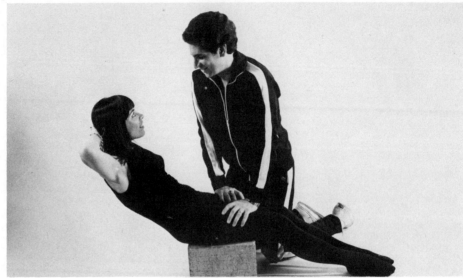

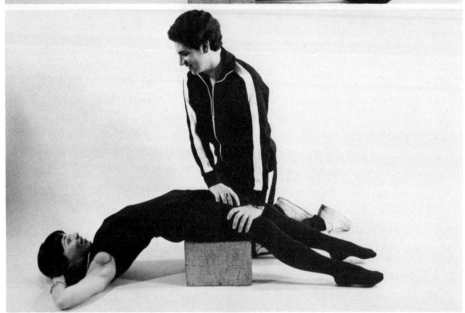

118

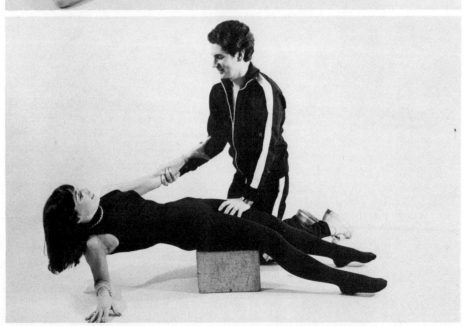

172. Roll down off bench, pull to sit up

Do this in turns. One of you sit on a low bench with your buttocks at the back edge. Your partner should hold your thighs as you lower your torso toward the floor, your hands clasped behind your neck. (See illustrations on previous page.) Stop when your shoulders touch the floor. *Don't* try to do a sit up; you might hurt your lower back. Instead, take your partner's hand, and both pull until you reach a sitting position. Repeat 4 times and change places with your partner.

14. Crab lift

Sit on the floor with your legs apart and knees bent. Lean back and place your hands behind you out to both sides, fingertips pointing back. Lift your body off the floor, making stomach, thighs, and chest nearly level, forming a square with your arms and calves as the sides and the floor as the base. Hold this position for 4 seconds, then relax, returning to the original position. Do 6 times.

173. On table—leg-lifts

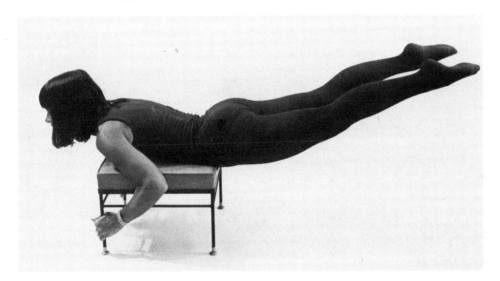

Place your torso in a prone position across the top of a low table or bench, and let your legs hang down to the floor. Using your hands for stability and balance, hold onto the table or bench and lift both of your legs into the air and straighten them out behind you. Lift them as high as you can, and hold the position for 4 seconds; then relax. Do 6 times.

174. Sitting—knees to floor

Sit on the floor. Bend your knees, placing the soles of your feet together, grasping your ankles with your hands, your elbows resting on your knees. With your elbows, press your knees to the floor as far down as they will go; then release. Do 12 times.

175. Overhead back-stretch

Lie supine and bring your bent knees over your torso. Slowly straighten your legs up into the air. Bring your buttocks off the floor and your legs down 119

(cont'd)

over your face, trying to touch your toes to the floor beyond your head. Go as far as you comfortably can, hold the position for 4 seconds, and then return to the original supine position, bending your knees as you lower your legs. Do 4 times.

82. Up goes the leg

Recline on your right side, leaning on your right elbow and forearm. Bend your left leg at the knee and bring it up toward your shoulder. With your left hand, grab the inside of your left foot, and slowly straighten your left leg as high as you can without pain. Pull your straight left leg toward your left shoulder 4 times and release. Do 4 times; then reverse sides.

25. Standing—pelvic tilt

Stand with feet apart, and bend your knees slightly, place your hands either on your thighs or your hips. Without moving your shoulders, push your bottom out; then draw it under and tighten your abdominals. Do this 8 to 16 times, being careful not to move your legs or shoulders.

162. On knees—pelvic tilt

Kneel down, resting your weight on your knees, shins, and insteps and keep your legs slightly apart. Without moving your shoulders, push your bottom out and then tuck it under, contracting your stomach muscles. Do 12 times.

27. Back—arch and flatten

Lie supine, and bend your knees to a 90-degree angle, keeping your feet flat on the floor. With your upper back and bottom on the floor, gently arch your lower back. Then flatten it, pressing it against the floor, and hold the position for 4 seconds. Repeat the entire exercise 6 times.

176. Supine—hip-lift

Lie supine, and bend your knees, keeping your feet flat on the floor and your arms at your sides with your palms on the floor. Lift your buttocks and push your hips up toward the ceiling. Hold for 4 seconds; then slowly lower your buttocks to the floor. Repeat 6 times.

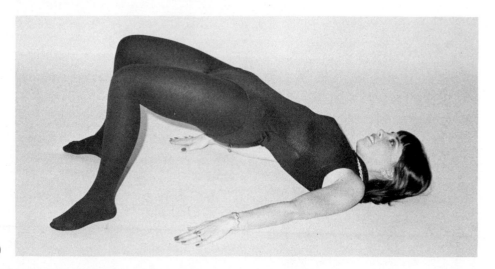

6. Prone—leg-lifts

Lie prone, resting your chin on folded arms. Keeping your hipbones on the floor, raise your right leg without bending your knee. Hold your leg in the air for 2 seconds; then lower it. Raise your left leg in the same manner, and repeat 16 times.

177. Bottoms up

Lie prone with your legs stretched out behind you, and rest your chin on your folded arms. Raise your buttocks in the air by drawing your knees up toward your stomach, and hold the position for 4 seconds before returning to the outstretched position. Repeat 6 times.

178. Prone—leg-kick and stretch

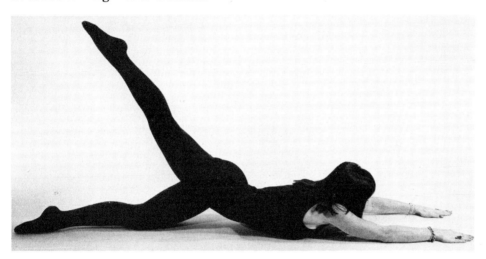

Lie prone with your arms stretched out straight above your head in front of you, resting your chin on the floor. Raise your straight right leg as high as possible and lift your hip off the floor. Hold your leg in the lifted position, stretching it out as far as you can for 4 seconds; then return your straight leg to the floor. Alternate legs, and repeat 12 times.

28. Prone—tighten and release

Lie in a prone position, resting your forehead or your chin on folded arms. Tighten your abdominals, buttock muscles, inner thighs, and vaginal muscles. Hold the contractions for 4 seconds; then release. Repeat 6 times.

22. Bent-knee sit-ups

Sit on the floor with your knees bent, and anchor your feet under a couch, dresser, or piece of sturdy furniture. Clasp your hands behind your neck, and from a sitting position slowly lie down. When your back is flat on the floor, sit up, keeping your hands clasped behind your neck. Come up with a rounded back; straighten your back only when you have reached the final sitting position. Start with 5 and work up to whatever is comfortable.

1. Back flat—leg-lower

Lie supine, and bring your knees over your chest, straightening your legs so that they form a 90-degree angle with your torso and the floor. Keeping the

121

(cont'd)

small of your back pressed firmly against the floor, slowly lower your legs *only* as far as you can without your back rising off the floor. (If you feel your back rising, you have lowered your legs too far.) When you reach that point, hold the position for 4 seconds; then release by bending your knees over your chin. Rest and repeat 4 times. *Never* lower your legs all the way to the floor, that will cause back strain.

179. Shoulder stand—bicycle

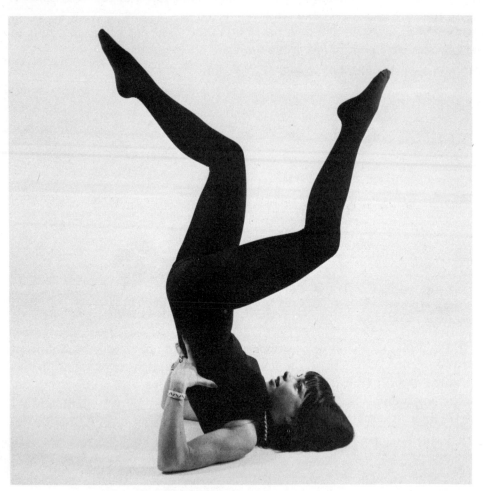

Lie supine with your legs stretched out and your arms at your sides. Bend your knees, and then slowly raise both legs over your head. Resting your weight on your shoulders, bend your arms, keeping your upper arms on the floor, and use your hands to support your lower back. Slowly straighten your torso and your legs into the air and hold this position for 2 seconds. Slowly move your legs in a circular motion as if you were riding a bicycle. Make 16 rotations; then slowly return to the original supine position.

180. Shoulder stand—knee-bend and stretch

Lie supine with your legs stretched out and your arms at your sides. Bend your knees and slowly raise both legs over your head. Resting your weight on your shoulders, bend your arms, keeping your upper arms on the floor, and

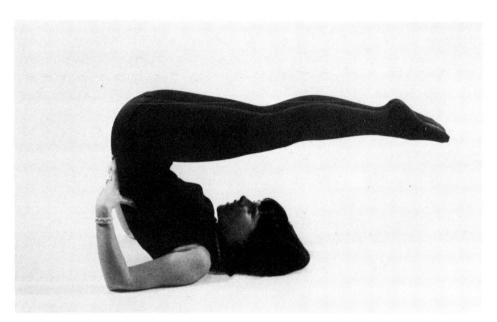

place your hands on your lower back for support. Slowly straighten your body and your legs into the air and, hold the position for 2 seconds. Slowly bend your knees down to your nose; then straighten your legs over your face, parallel to the floor. Hold the position for 2 seconds; then bend your knees again. Repeat the movements 4 times; then slowly return to the original position.

181. Shoulder stand—one-leg–stretch

Lie supine with your legs stretched out and your arms at your sides. Bend your knees, slowly raising both legs over your head. Resting your weight on your shoulders, bend your arms, keeping your upper arms on the floor, and place your hands on your lower back for support. Slowly straighten your body and your legs vertically into the air, and hold the position for 2 seconds. Slowly lower your straight right leg down over your face, keeping your straight left leg up in the air. Hold the position for 2 seconds, and raise your right leg again. Slowly lower your straight left leg over your face, keeping your right leg up in the air and hold the position for 2 seconds. Return left leg to a vertical position and repeat 4 times. Slowly return to the original position.

182. Split

Get down on your hands and knees. Lean your weight on your left knee, and place your right foot between your hands. Slide your right foot forward until your right leg is straight out in front of you. Leaning your weight on both hands, slowly straighten your left leg out behind you and lower your crotch toward the floor as far as you can without pain. You will feel a pulling sensation on the top of your left leg and the back of your right. Hold the position for 4 seconds, and return to the original position. Alternate legs now, and then repeat the exercise 4 times, always using your arms to balance your weight.

183. Push-ups

Get down in a push-up position, supporting yourself on your palms and the balls of your feet. Keeping your body straight, slowly lower yourself, letting your chest touch the floor first. Once down, relax. Rise any way you can and assume the push-up position again. As you lower yourself, count to 6 and do 4 times. When you are strong enough, you will be able to raise your straight body in the push-up position.

90. Run in place

Do just that for 150 to 500 steps.

6

Long Day's Journey Out of Stress and Tension

Some of us are more susceptible to anxiety than others, but everyone is plagued by it to varying degrees in our high-pressured, success-oriented culture. Tranquilizers, particularly Valium and Librium, provide temporary relief when used according to a doctor's prescription. Less efficient but more dangerous are three commonly misused "drugs": alcohol, tobacco, and a super-abundant diet.

A certain amount of anxiety motivates us to complete tasks and achieve goals. Anxiety originates in childhood, usually with one's parents, continues throughout education, and then into a profession. No matter what the job, most of us are faced with pressure to succeed, to earn enough money, and to find outlets for our aggressions. Those pressures, while they motivate us, also increase our anxieties.

Those who perform well seem to have an inner calm, what Hemingway referred to as "grace under pressure." We all have different levels of tolerance for pressure and its partner, anxiety. When the flame of pressure is turned up too high, most people suffer a variety of symptoms, ranging from mild irritability to flashes of anger or a sense of depression when the pressure leaves one feeling helpless. Others, dreading what lies ahead, may attempt to douse the fire with alcohol before it turns into a conflagration, postponing the inevitable by retreating into a non-functioning state. Still others may calm themselves with the aid of tranquilizers. Tranquilizers have certain values, but other depressants, such as alcohol, are self-defeating and harmful to health as well.

When anxious, many of us overeat and become obese. Obesity results in self-loathing, which further increases anxiety, which in turn fuels compulsive overeating, and thus goes the vicious cycle.

During anxiety, most of us cannot relax our muscles and don't even try; they remain tense and contracted, which often leads to aches and pains, if not debilitating muscle spasms. Fortunately, it is possible to learn to relax, to fight off the manifestations of stress and tension. Even from our cat, we have learned lessons. She does not keep her tension bottled up; instead, she races around the living room (not altogether different from jogging), hisses if antagonized, then finds a comfortable shelf on which to stretch out her elegantly sinuous body. Her muscles are relaxed, and so is she. We, on the other hand, are endowed with particularly human qualities, which, if properly utilized, can make our lives bearable and healthy.

Backed into a Corner

At Suzy Prudden Studios, we have seen many cases of lower-back pain caused by a combination of tension and weak lower backs. In *Back-Ache, Stress and Tension*, Dr. Hans Kraus wrote, "Clinical studies show that more than 80 percent of all back-pain cases are caused by underexercise."

What often occurs is quite simple: Weak lower-back muscles tense too quickly during prolonged periods of stress and tension. When lower-back pain strikes, it can be excruciating, forcing the victim to spend days lying supine, the slightest movement causing pain. Often, in fact, it is a quick movement which sends the already tense muscles into spasm. The muscles contract so tightly that some people have been locked into angular positions, unable to stand up straight or sit down.

If you have not yet begun our back exercises, and you have suffered a muscle spasm, lie supine on a hard surface with your knees bent. Then see a back specialist, preferably one who doesn't see surgery as the answer.

If you have a weak lower back, do all you can to avoid injury. Even if you have a strong lower back, you must be careful. When you lift something, particularly a heavy object, never bend from the waist or hips. Always bend your legs at the knees, take hold of the object, and slowly straighten up. Never make sudden movements which can wrench muscles.

Exercise can prevent lower-back pain, or at least reduce its subsequent intensity. Even if you have a strong lower back, lack of regular exercise, lack of sleep, and prolonged periods of stress and tension can result in pain. You may not be able to escape difficult situations, but you can certainly get enough sleep and begin to exercise your lower back, if only for five minutes a day. At the end of this chapter you will find special back exercises which are helpful.

Since the back is such a sensitive area, we suggest you check with your doctor before you begin exercising.

Slowly, try to touch your toes without bending your knees. If you cannot, and if you feel pain in your back and legs, you have tense hamstrings and a tense back, as well. Start with our stretchercises, and wait a week or two before going on to our other exercises.

If you do little or nothing to relax those tense muscles, the stress and tension of everyday life will make their condition worse. People who are required to sit at desks day after day are especially susceptible to weak, tense lower-back muscles. Legs and shoulders are other vulnerable areas.

In overcrowded urban centers, men and women are packed together with few opportunities to release tension in natural settings. In many cities, people are frightened to break into a run, wary of being mistaken for a mugger or chased by an unleashed dog. During certain hours, the streets are too crowded to accommodate anyone who does not care to shuffle along in an anonymous crowd. In such environments, millions suffer the effects of stress and tension. Only those who are fortunate enough to enjoy the benefits of physical labor can truly *work* off the noxious effects of our society.

The rest of us will have to settle for exercise, which requires strong motivations and an ongoing commitment.

No Sleep for the Weary

Another, even more common, result of stress and tension is insomnia. Millions rely on sleeping pills of varying strengths, though most of us could fall asleep naturally if we could reduce our levels of stress and tension.

If one reaches the early evening of each day with a head full of problems, then one will probably gobble down dinner (causing indigestion), drink too much alcohol (deadening the brain), watch too much television (alienating one's mate), and then go to bed only to toss and turn most of the night.

Through our work with adult students at Suzy Prudden Studios, we have developed a series of relaxercises which help prepare you for sleep. They are all at the end of this chapter. The relaxercises teach you how to drain off excess tension and stretch your muscles so that they will be ready for sleep.

The next step is simple, almost a kind of self-hypnosis. It begins with getting into a comfortable position conducive to sleep; then, through the power of suggestion, you lull your body into deeper relaxation. Start by telling yourself that your face is relaxed, your eyelids are closing, your lips are relaxing, tension is leaving your neck. All the while, your breathing should be slow, deep, and steady. Move down your entire body, relaxing every part of it, slowly and gently. Next try to concentrate on one word, any word, as long as it has no negative connotations. All of your energies, both conscious and subconscious, will become focused on the word you choose. If a single word doesn't work, choose an object or a person, perhaps someone you have always wanted to know. Choose something with pleasant connotations that can take you off into wish-fulfillment dreams.

Pass the Fashion Plate

The way you dress can either increase or decrease one's tensions. It is important to dress for comfort as well as for good looks rather than for good looks only. Throughout the years, there have been many fashions that have contributed to tightly contracted muscles (platform shoes and high heels) or to inadequate circulation (chokers, tight pants, and tight skirts). We suggest you dress in clothing that permits your blood to circulate freely and doesn't alter the natural positions of your muscles or vital organs.

When you buy a shirt, choose one half a size too large. If you have to wear a tie, don't knot it around your throat as a hangman would. If your neck is free to move as it should, you will diminish the likelihood of upper-back pain, stiff necks, and even migraines, common hazards in our society today.

Every day you see examples of people warding off the additional tension that results from tight clothing. Men with ulcers or stomach cramps invariably loosen their belts. Shoes which pinch the feet are often slipped off feet hidden beneath a desk. Even the elastic on tight socks can decrease circulation, causing feet to fall asleep. Garters can be even worse; they usually cut into muscles as well as into veins. If you wear any elastic clothing, be sure it isn't so tight that it inhibits circulation, tensing muscles needlessly.

One of the worst offenders is the girdle: It is tight all over, has a negative effect on circulation, and it does the work of muscles, causing unused muscles to fall into even deeper disuse. As a general rule, avoid a girdle and use nature's girdle—your muscles. If properly exercised, they do a superb job.

The best shoes are the most comfortable ones, those which let your feet breathe and move freely. Probably the best example of such a shoe is the ancient Roman sandal. Of course, they cannot be worn in all forms of weather and to all occasions. However, there are many varieties of comfortable shoe styles on the market which are sufficiently attractive for any time and any place.

Just as most parents no longer wrap their infants in swaddling clothes, so adults should not wrap themselves in clothes that hamper muscles and diminish circulation. Life imposes enough stresses and tensions on us without our adding to them.

If You Hatha Time, We Hatha Yoga

In the last few years, yoga has enjoyed a vogue among many people who rarely, if ever, seriously exercised. And that, undoubtedly, has contributed to its popularity, for it seems to require no exertion. In addition, it took its place alongside transcendental meditation and other manifestations of a mushrooming interest in Eastern mysticism.

Though yoga may, indeed, be enjoyable, it is hardly one of the more energetic isotonic exercises. Voluntary muscles are not quickly and repeatedly contracted and relaxed, and you are not left breathing hard and fast. If you have sufficient energy and stamina to jog for several miles, you will probably not find yoga a vigorous enough activity. In fact, many health-conscious individuals feel a daily need to expend hundreds of calories in an endurance sport and might only find yoga useful to completely relax after they have completed their more vigorous activities. Still, a small amount of yoga integrated into your daily fitness program leads to an extra sense of relaxation and tranquility.

It should be apparent that we do not regard yoga as an alternative to vigorous isotonic exercises, but we do believe that it has its place for those so inclined. For those who wish to meditate, yoga may be an apt corollary. We ourselves utilize various yoga principles at Suzy Prudden Studios, but only as an integral part of an invigorating physical fitness program.

Each yoga position consists of three basic movements, collectively known as *Asanas*. First, you assume a particular position; second, you maintain that position as statically as possible while you concentrate, breathing slowly and deeply; third, you return slowly and gracefully to the original position. All this is done with precise control and a kind of fluidity.

After you have completed each step of an *Asana*, you are usually instructed to lie supine and enjoy the depths of pure relaxation. The entire process gently tenses, then relaxes, various muscles. In addition to its relaxing effects, yoga is regarded as extremely beneficial to circulation, positively affecting high blood pressure. Yoga even helps to alleviate migraines and constipation. Because yoga is directed toward the goal of serenity, it markedly develops the powers of concentration. The benefits of that are manifold and can be applied in many areas, ranging from your occupation to insomnia.

Because most of us have hectic schedules, evenings and weekends provide the best times in which to perform Hatha Yoga. Proper clothing is as important as the proper atmosphere, so wear what makes you feel most comfortable while exercising.

At the end of this chapter, you will find a few basic *Asanas* which we believe can be incorporated into your daily fitness program. We suggest you use them as relaxercises after you have done the more vigorous exercises. If you don't have enough time for the *Asanas*, we suggest a few minutes on the weekends or before you go to sleep at night.

It Doesn't Melt Away

We know people who emerge from saunas and steam baths as happily as if they had just completed psychoanalysis. We have seen others who have barely (no pun intended) oozed out, eyes glassed over, mouths desperate for an icy glass of water. Saunas and steam baths are salubrious for some, deleterious for others.

Many elderly people should stay out of saunas and steam baths unless their doctors have given them permission; those who have heart conditions should stay out, too. In fact, the warning list is long, including anyone with high blood pressure, diabetes, anyone taking a drug that causes drowsiness, and anyone who has had too much to drink. Sleeping pills or tranquilizers make saunas *verboten* to the consumer. The same applies to any of the "hard drugs." Anticoagulants or antihistamines make steam baths and saunas worse than merely uncomfortable.

It takes very little time or effort to check with your physician, and we advise it as a matter of course. Now that we have dealt out the appropriate cautions, we hope there are still a few of you who may enjoy and benefit from either a sauna or a steam bath.

Once inside, make yourself comfortable and relax. If you forgot to do your push-ups, don't do them in such a hot house, unless, of course, you want to be carried out on a stretcher. Don't jog around in a little circle, and leave your jump rope outside. Sitting in a sauna or steam bath is one of the few non-activities which provides an opportunity for tired, tense muscles to completely relax. Enjoy the luxury of doing nothing; yet realize that you are doing something superb for yourself. Wait at least an hour after you have eaten before you go inside; however, it is perfectly all right to imbibe liquids (nonalcoholic, of course) either before, during, or after, since the heat makes you perspire profusely, creating a feeling of dehydration.

Be careful not to stay in a sauna or steam bath too long, especially when you first start using one. We suggest you consult your doctor about the appropriate amount of time for you since this varies from person to person. Generally speaking, we recommend that you start with just a few minutes and gradually increase to the limit established by your doctor.

The heat of a sauna can have a positive effect on your circulation and will also precipitate water loss, causing a temporary reduction in your weight. Best of all, it will relax muscles which are crying out for warmth and relaxation.

In professional health clubs, many clients have a massage or a rubdown after a sauna or a steam bath. Massage relaxes tense muscles, while stimulating the flow of blood through them, causing a surge of new vitality.

The overall effect of saunas and steam baths is a significant reduction of stress and tension. You emerge feeling more youthful, more vigorous, and more healthy than before.

Warm to hot baths are available to almost everyone, and most people find them relaxing, particularly after an invigorating workout.

Warmth, in varying degrees, relaxes your muscles, and the longer you stay in a tub, the greater is your sense of relaxation. However, relaxation can be carried too far, and the happily relaxed bather can easily fall asleep. If you are pooped, don't even get into a tub, and if you feel yourself becoming increasingly drowsy while bathing, get thee to dry land.

The average tub of water can be made even more relaxing by the addition of a whirlpool device. A whirlpool circulates the water, giving the bather a feeling of being gently massaged. Heat and massage are ancient and valuable remedies for tired, tense muscles. In drugstores throughout the world you can buy chemical compounds which create a sensation of heat when rubbed on the skin. They are commonly used to treat aching joints, as well as tense muscles. And since the installation of household electricity, people have been happily applying heating pads to sore areas.

Re-create and Recreate

Childhood is best remembered as a time of endless recreation, a time when the sun set too early and rose too late. It was rarely, if ever, a time for prolonged introspection, and fights were settled quickly for the sake of having fun.

It's difficult for any mature adult to re-create the days that now exist in a fuzzy state of memory. Those days are probably best left where they are, charming in their distance. But there are aspects of children at play which no adult should ever forget. In play comes an opportunity to avoid self-doubt and to build self-confidence.

In New York's Central Park, a New Yorker can see groups of professional men and women engaged in a variety of sporting events, from touch football to softball. With a delight that could easily rival any child's, they compete with one another in a concentrated effort to reduce the stress and tensions of their worlds.

There are other forms of recreation, such as jogging, tennis, and squash, which can serve as tension breakers. For us, the best antidote to tension and fatigue is some pleasurable physical activity. We especially enjoy an evening of dancing and find it a rejuvenating experience. It really doesn't matter what you choose, as long as you choose something that gives you a lift, physically and mentally. Being tired or not having enough time are no excuses for inactivity. Long walks are excellent for relaxation, and many people utilize the time for thinking and making decisions. You can play squash or tennis at any hour of the day. You can jog to the office or home. You can swim so many laps that tension will drain out of your muscles.

Though our highly mechanized society is a nearly endless source of stress and tension, it does provide us with enough leisure time to be either soft or strong, unfit or vigorous. Recreation provides us with wonderful opportunities to re-create the best aspects of childhood and adolescence; it is a form of therapy that helps to make us all more vital and youthful.

Many people wait for weekends to enjoy themselves; others, less patient, wait until they leave their offices. However, you can easily fit recreation into lunch hours. Have a container of yogurt or a salad, and then go to a neighborhood health club for an exercise class, a swim, or a game of squash. The afternoon will go by quickly, because you will have the energy to make those hours productive. You'll be adding measurably to your physical fitness, and you may advance your career at the same time. Many very successful people alternate work with play in order to maintain high levels of energy, enabling them to reach their goals with breath to spare.

Earlier, we described how you can put yourself into a state of relaxation conducive to sleep. That exercise not only works for insomniacs but for many others who find themselves particularly tense in various situations. And it works in the privacy of your office, on an airplane, and before getting out of bed.

At Suzy Prudden Studios, we conclude all exercise classes by putting our students into a similar state of relaxation. Having vigorously exercised for fifty short minutes, the students are asked to stand and shake out their limbs. Then they are instructed to stand on their toes and stretch their arms as high above their heads as they can. They feel the tips of their fingers reaching out as if trying to tickle infinity. Then they release the stretching position, allowing their muscles to relax. Having stretched and relaxed, the students then recline on their backs. Their muscles have been given a thorough work-out; their bodies are tingling with vigor and strength.

They close their eyes, the music is turned off, and only the sounds of breathing prevail. Beginning slowly and steadily, almost in a whisper, the instructor says, "Breathe in, now out, deeply in, now out." A rhythm of relaxed but controlled breathing is established, continuing until the students have cooled off. Then they are told to let their faces relax, to let all their facial muscles go limp. The routine goes something like this: "Slowly inhale, now slowly exhale, that's right. Again, slowly inhale, exhale. Let your face

131

relax, feel all of it is muscles going limp; let your face fall to the side. Inhale. Exhale. Feel your neck relaxing, now your shoulders, your upper arms, your lower arms, your hands, and fingertips. Inhale. Exhale. Inhale. Exhale. Let your pectoral muscles relax. Let your stomach and lower back relax. Inhale slowly. Exhale slowly. Feel your pelvic area relax, feel your buttocks and thighs relax. Your knees bend slightly, and they relax, too. Your calf muscles are relaxing, your ankles and their tendons are relaxing. You can feel the bottoms of your feet relaxing, and even your toes seem to be relaxing. Inhale slowly, and now exhale slowly. That's right. Gently and slowly inhale again, and exhale, inhale and exhale."

We suggest that you repeat this entire process as we do in our classes in order to feel marvelously refreshed and relaxed. After the second time, stretch your arms above your head while keeping them on the floor. Stretch harder and try to make your body grow longer. Point your toes and stretch your fingertips until you feel you cannot go any further. Then release. Let go suddenly, and just lie supine in a fully relaxed position. Don't get up immediately; you may get dizzy. Let your body adjust and slowly get up, sitting for a minute and then standing.

Of course, only a modified version of this routine can be done in your office or on a plane, but it can and should be done. You'll feel clearheaded and energetic; at ease and close to a state of serenity.

Stretching, by itself, especially in the morning when you wake up, relaxes your body and gives you a marvelous feeling of coordination and flexibility with which to face the day.

The Rules of the Game

1. The point of this book, and this chapter in particular, is that you should be good to yourself, physically, mentally, and emotionally. If you are physically fit, able to find adequate releases for tension, you will be good to yourself—and a highly esteemed partner to someone else, as well.

If you find yourself saying "But I don't have the time; I have too much work to do," you may be a workaholic. Workaholism can become a self-destructive form of behavior. The compulsion to complete tasks that preoccupy all of the waking hours is only one system of repression; the workaholic is indulging in a form of self-punishment in order to alleviate anxiety about a repressed concern. If such an individual refuses psychotherapy, some help can be gained through the physical therapy of a pleasurable activity. For instance, if you are married to a workaholic, you may be able to persuade such a person to spend an evening dancing or an afternoon at a health club, in that way reducing tensions while refreshing the exhausted body.

2. Refresh yourself. If your problems are creating overwhelming anxieties, slow down, get out, and refresh yourself. Try to relegate your responsibilities to someone else, at least long enough for a change of pace, a different scene. Remove yourself from the jungle of problems and do something to occupy your mind and body pleasantly—anything from a long walk to a chat with a thoughtful friend. Though your problems may still be there when you return,

you will feel refreshed enough to deal with them with a vigorous, new outlook.

3. Center your ego. The poet e.e. cummings claimed that he had never met anyone who was not egocentric. He was not being critical; he was merely remarking on a human condition.

If your ego is properly located, if you center it, you can see things as they are. The person who neither overreacts nor underreacts, but simply reacts realistically will not suffer the deleterious effects of stress and tension.

We all have to bear a certain number of minor indignities, but the self-serving wise individual knows which situations to ignore and which to confront. Remember that you are the victim of your own pride and prejudice.

4. Unmask tragedy. Don't elevate every minor misfortune into a tragedy. Take disappointment in your stride—and take time out for laughter.

5. Keep your problems out of bed. Problems should be dealt with during the day. If you postpone problems until bedtime, a restful night's sleep will be an improbability.

Tranquilizers can diminish the size of those problems, but they can also make you a less spirited lover. Try our relaxercises first. They'll leave you refreshed and ready for love, and for a good night's sleep; you may even find that you no longer need tranquilizers.

On a physical level, a firm mattress is a must for the support you need to avoid aching muscles and lower-back pain in the morning.

6. Never eat and run. Eat slowly in a pleasant, relaxed atmosphere; listen to pleasant music, enjoy good conversation.

7. Relaxercise. No matter how busy you may think you are, you should never be too busy to relax through exercising. Our relaxercises will ease tension and invigorate tired muscles, enabling you to enjoy life as fully as possible.

SHOULDERS AND NECK

4. Prone—arm-lifts

Lie prone with your chin on the floor and your arms stretched out in front of you. Lift your right arm into the air as high as you can, keeping it beside your ear and keeping your chin on the floor. Lower your right arm; then lift your left arm in the same manner. Repeat 16 times.

12. The swim

Stand with your feet apart and bend forward from the hips. Move your arms in a swimming motion, making complete circular movements. Each arm should circle 16 times.

89. Arm-swing

Stand with your feet apart and your arms stretched out to the sides, level with your shoulders. Swing both arms, first to the left and then to the right, following the movement with your nose. Throughout, keep your hips from moving. Do 16 times.

18. The back of my hand

This exercise can be done with feet either together or apart. Keeping your left arm at your side, raise your right arm, bending it at the elbow. Place the back of your right hand against your right cheek. Swing your arm, stretching your hand backwards and away from your face until your arm is as straight as a backstroker's. Do the same with your left hand and arm, leaving your right at your side. Do each arm 8 times.

13A. Shoulders back and forth

Standing with your feet together and your arms at your sides, push your shoulders forward, rounding them and your back. Reverse the movement, pushing your shoulders back as far as possible. Do 16 times.

13B. The shrug

After finishing the exercise above, try to raise your shoulders up to your ears. Lower shoulders and lift your head, stretching your neck. Do this one 16 times.

86. Shoulder circle

Stand with your feet slightly apart and your arms at your sides. Tighten your abdominals and slowly push your shoulders forward; then lift your shoulders up to your ears and slowly stretch your shoulders back as far as you can. Finally, lower your shoulders to the original position. Repeat the forward circular motion 8 times; then reverse the direction. Repeat 8 times.

UPPER BACK

184. Round back to stretch—chest-thrust to straight-leg crab

Sit with your legs bent at the knees and your feet flat on the floor. Keeping your legs together, clasp your shins with your hands, round your back, and tuck your head down. Tighten your abdominals and hold for 4 seconds. Stretch your legs out in front of you and put your hands on the floor behind

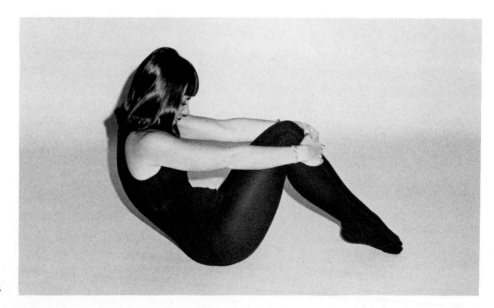

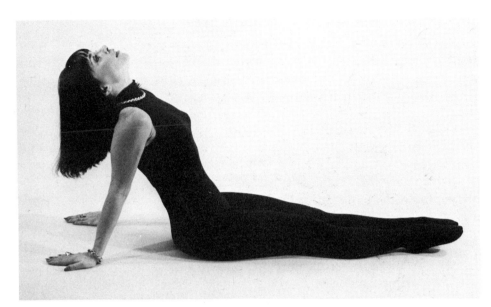

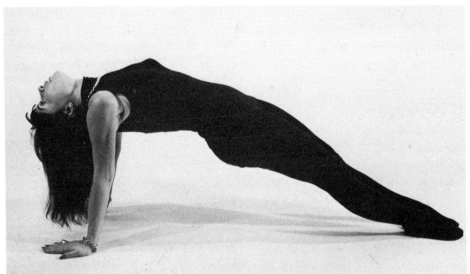

you. Thrust your chest up into the air, arching your back and straightening your legs. Lift your bottom off the floor, thrusting your hips into the air. Hold for 4 seconds, and return to a sitting position. Repeat 4 times.

65. Pushing marbles with your nose

Get down on your hands and knees and stretch your arms out as far as you can in front of you, resting your bottom on your heels. Move your torso forward, keeping your head close to the floor as if pushing an imaginary marble with your nose. Your head will pass your arms which will be bent at the elbows. After your nose has gone forward as far as possible, raise your head, straightening your arms, and push your entire torso upward. Return to the original position, your bottom resting on your heels, and repeat the exercise 4 times.

101. On knees—lean back, thrust forward

Get down on your hands and knees and stretch your straight arms out in front of you as far as you can, resting your buttocks on your heels. Push your torso forward, supporting yourself on straight arms and legs bent at the knees. Return to original position. Repeat 8 times.

21. Paint the wall

Get down on your hands and knees. As if you had a can of paint on your right side, and a paintbrush and a wall to paint on your left, reach with your left hand under your right side, and then swing your left hand back out toward the right, lifting it as high as you can. Do 4 times; then change arms.

87. Overhead arm-stretch

Stand with your feet together and stretch your arms up straight above your head. Bend your right leg at the knee and stretch your right arm higher above your head, as hard and as far as you can. Hold for 4 seconds. Release your right arm, keeping it above your head, and straighten your right leg. Bend your left leg at the knee and stretch your left arm higher above your head, as hard and as far as you can. Hold for 4 seconds. Release your left arm, keeping it above your head, and straighten your left leg. Repeat series 8 times.

19. Airplane stretch

Standing with your feet apart, bring your arms up to shoulder height. Bend them at the elbows until your fingers touch in front of you. Quickly bring your elbows back as far as you can; then return them to the starting position with your hands in front of you. Straighten your arms out to the sides, keeping them at shoulder height, and turn your palms upward. Return to the original position, and repeat 12 times.

85. Airplane stretch and circle

Stand with your feet apart, fingertips of both hands touching in front of your chest, elbows out at your sides at shoulder height. Gently bring your elbows back behind you as far as you can; then return to the original position. Straighten your arms out in front of you, then raise them straight up, then back, and then down, making a full circular motion with your arms. Return your arms to the original position, elbows bent and fingertips touching in front of your chest. Repeat entire exercise 8 times; then reverse circular motion. Repeat again 8 times.

5. Corner push-ups

At a distance of about 2 to 3 feet, face a corner of a room and stand with your feet together. Place your palms against each wall of the corner with your arms at shoulder height. Keeping your body straight, lean forward, bringing your face and chest as close to the corner as possible; then push off, back to an erect position. Repeat 8 times, keeping your elbows at shoulder height at all times.

LOWER BACK

185. Leg-to-chest back-press

Lie supine with your legs stretched out, your arms at your sides, and the back of your head on the floor. Raise your head, looking down toward your stomach, and lift your right leg, bending it at the knee, and then raising it over your chest. Clasp your hands around your right shin, just under the knee, and pull your right leg against your chest while you press your lower back against the floor. Hold for 4 seconds; then alternate legs. Repeat 8 times.

6. Prone—leg-lifts

Lie prone, resting your chin on folded arms. Keeping your hipbones on the floor, raise your right leg without bending the knee. Hold your leg in the air for 2 seconds; then lower it. Raise your left leg in the same manner. Repeat 16 times.

1. Back flat—leg-lower

Lie supine. Bring your knees up over your chest, and then straighten your legs so that they form a 90-degree angle with your torso and the floor. Keeping the small of your back pressed firmly against the floor, slowly lower your legs *only* as far as you can without your back rising off the floor. (If you feel your back rising, you have lowered your legs too far.) When you reach that point, hold the position for 4 seconds; then release by bending your knees over your chest. Rest and repeat 4 times. *Never* lower your legs all the way to the floor, that will cause back strain.

27. Back—arch and flatten

Lie supine. Bend your knees to a 90-degree angle and keep your feet flat on the floor. With your upper back and bottom on the floor, gently arch your lower back. Then flatten it, gently pressing it against the floor. Hold the flattened position for 4 seconds, and repeat the entire exercise 6 times.

61. The metronome

Lie supine. Raise your legs, bending your knees up over your chest. Bend your arms, resting them on the floor with your hands beside your shoulders. Press the small of your back against the floor, and slowly lower your bent legs to the left, trying to keep both shoulders on the floor. Lift your bent legs off the floor, bringing them back over your chest and pressing the small of your back against the floor. Slowly lower your legs to the right side, and repeat 16 times.

63. The feline

Get down on your hands and knees. Slowly lower your head and round your back, lifting it upward while you suck in your stomach. Hold for 3 seconds; then raise your head and slowly lower your back, letting it sag in the middle. Repeat 8 times.

137

22. Bent-knee sit-ups

Sit on the floor with your knees bent and anchor your feet under a couch, dresser, or piece of sturdy furniture. Clasp your hands behind your neck, and, from a sitting position, slowly lie down. When your back is flat on the floor, sit up, keeping your hands clasped behind your neck. Come up with a rounded back and straighten it when you have reached the final sitting position. Start with 5 and work up to whatever is comfortable.

23. Bicycle

Sit on the floor and lean back on your elbows and forearms. Raise your legs, moving them as if you were peddling a bicycle. As you bring one leg up over your chest, your other leg should stretch straight out. At no time should either of your legs touch the floor. Do 16 times.

24. On elbows—knees to chest, straighten, and circle

Lean back on your elbows and forearms, and bend your knees up over your chest. Release and straighten your legs straight up; then slowly separate them. As they separate, they will lower, forming a circle in the air. Bring your legs together about 4 to 6 inches off the floor, and hold the position for 3 seconds. Repeat the exercise 4 times, each week adding an additional rotation. If you feel pain in your lower back at any time, stop. Do this exercise after a few weeks when your muscles are stronger and your body in better shape.

176. Supine hip-lift

Lie supine. Bend your knees with your feet flat on the floor, and rest your arms at your sides with your palms on the floor. Lift your buttocks off the floor, pushing your hips up toward the ceiling. Hold the position for 4 seconds; then slowly lower your buttocks to the floor. Repeat 6 times.

186. Supine—knees bent, rest

Lie supine with your legs bent at the knees and your feet flat on the floor. Place your arms at your sides, and gently press the small of your back against the floor. Hold for 4 seconds; then relax your stomach and lower-back muscles.

ALL IN ONE

187. Round back and straighten

Sit on the floor with your legs bent at the knees and your feet flat on the floor. Keeping your legs together, clasp your shins with your hands, round your back, and tuck your head down. Tighten your abdominals and hold the position for 4 seconds. Don't tighten your shoulders. Slowly straighten your back, pressing your chest and stomach toward your thighs, lifting your face toward the ceiling. Hold for 4 seconds and release. Repeat 4 times. (See illustrations on following page.)

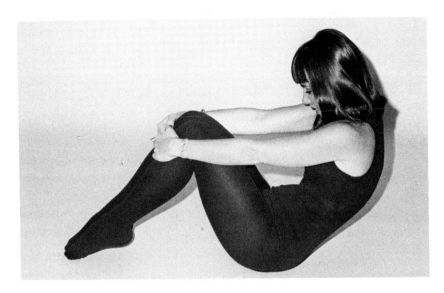

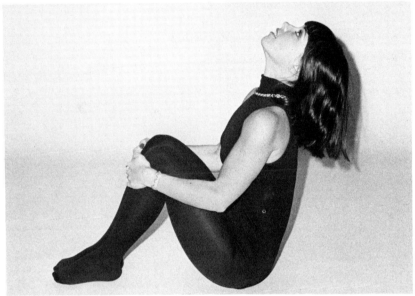

LEGS

31. Half knee-bend, heel-down

Stand with your feet together and your arms stretched out straight in front of you. Bend your knees as if doing a deep knee-bend, but only go halfway down. Keep your heels and the rest of your feet flat on the floor. Do 16 times.

36. Heel-up

Stand with your feet together and your hands at your sides. Raise your right heel by going up onto the ball and toes of your right foot, and lean your weight on your left leg. Alternate from right foot to left foot, holding each position to a count of 3. Repeat alternations 16 times.

139

39. Curl feet and flatten

Stand with your feet together and your arms at your sides. Shift so that your weight is on the outside of your feet, and curl your toes under. Hold the position for 4 seconds; then return to a flat-footed stance. Do 8 times.

40. Toes stretch and release

You can do this exercise standing, sitting, or lying down, but be sure your feet are bare. Stretch and separate your toes, holding the position for 4 seconds before releasing your muscles. Repeat 10 times for each foot. Then curl your toes under and hold for 2 seconds to release all the tension in your foot. If your foot cramps, do the exercise 4 times only, and don't continue the exercise while your foot is cramped. Return to it later.

43. Knee-wag

Stand with your feet and knees together; slightly bend your knees and lean on the outer part of your right foot and the inner part of your left. Sway your knees to the right, then alternate the direction of your sway, move back and forth 16 times.

188. On elbow—knee-bend in front and straighten

Lie on your right side, leaning on your right elbow and forearm, with your left palm on the floor in front of your stomach. Keep your legs straight so that your body and legs form a straight line. Without moving your torso, bend your left knee and raise it up toward your chest. Straighten it out again, and bend and straighten 8 times; then roll over and repeat 8 times with your right leg.

189. On elbow—leg-bend to the side, straighten leg up and then lower

Lie on your right side, leaning on your right elbow and forearm and placing your left palm on the floor in front of your stomach. Keep your legs straight so that your body and legs form a straight line. Without moving your torso, turn your left leg so that the tops of your thigh, knee, shin, and foot face the ceiling. Bend your knee and raise it up toward your shoulder as high as you can. Then straighten your left leg up into the air. Slowly lower your straight left leg to your straight right leg, but don't rest it. Repeat 8 times, roll over, and do 8 times with your right leg.

49. Infinity leg-swing

Sit on the floor, lean back on your elbows and forearms, and stretch your legs out in front of you. Flex your right foot and lift it, turning it to the left. Cross it over your left leg until you can place your right big toe just beyond your left leg. Reverse the motion and bring your right foot back wide, turning the entire foot to the right. Repeat 8 times with each leg.

STRETCHERCISES

9. Sitting—forward bounce, legs straight, feet together

Sit on the floor with your legs straight out in front of you and your feet together. Hold your legs, pull your torso forward, and then release it backward. You should feel a stretching in the backs of your legs. Bounce forward and back 16 times with your toes pointed, then flex your feet so that your toes point up toward the ceiling, and bounce 16 times.

29. Sitting—side-to-side bounce, chin-to-toe, ear-to-knee

A. Sit on the floor with your legs moderately wide apart and stretched out straight. With both of your hands, hold your right knee and flex your right foot, stretching the calves and backs of the thighs. Keeping your head and chin up, push your torso forward, then back, and pretend to touch your toes with your chin. After 8 bounces, shift to your other leg, always keeping your chin up.

B. Remain in the position of the exercise above. Instead of leading with your chin, try to touch your ear to your knee without bending your knee. Do 8 times; then reverse legs.

8. Standing—forward bounce

Stand with your feet apart, your legs straight, and your hands clasped behind you. Bounce forward, bending at the hips, as low as you comfortably can without bending your knees. Keeping your arms straight, bring your hands up behind you as you bounce forward. Bounce 8 times forward, 8 times over the right leg, 8 times forward, 8 times over the left leg, and, finally, 8 times forward again.

30. Standing—toes on book, heel-lower

Stand with your feet together and the balls of the feet on the edge of a thick book (phone books are great). Slowly lower your heels to the floor; then raise yourself onto the balls of your feet again. Tighten your abdominals and buttock muscles to maintain your balance. Raise and lower your heels 16 times.

88. Side-to-side leg-stretch and bounce

Stand with your feet apart and your hands clasped behind your buttocks. Keeping your left foot pointed forward, turn your right foot out to point right, turning your body until it faces right. Do 4 half knee-bends on your right leg, keeping your left leg straight. Straighten your right leg and do 4 forward bounces over your right leg, raising your clasped hands up behind you as high as you can. Repeat the series 4 times. Return your right foot to the original position, and turn your left foot to the left. Repeat the exercise 4 times to the left.

58. Holding hands—side-to-side bounce

Stand with your feet together and place your hands on the fronts of your thighs. Bend your knees until your fingers touch the floor, keeping your arms straight. With your fingertips on the floor, straighten your legs, pushing your bottom into the air. Hold the position for 3 seconds; then return to the original upright position. Do 8 times.

82. Up goes the leg

Recline on the right side, leaning on your right elbow and forearm. Bend your left leg at the knee, and bring your knee up toward your shoulder. With your left hand, grab the inside of your left foot and slowly straighten your left leg up as high as you can without pain. Pull your straight left leg toward your left shoulder 4 times and release. Do 4 times; then reverse sides.

187. Round back and straighten

Sit on the floor with your legs bent at the knees and your feet flat on the floor. Keeping your legs together, clasp your shins with both your hands, round your back, and tuck your head down. Tighten your abdominals and hold the position for 12 seconds. Don't tighten your shoulders. Slowly straighten your back, pressing your chest and stomach toward your thighs while lifting your face toward the ceiling. Hold for 12 seconds and release. Repeat 4 times.

174. Sitting—knees to floor

Sit on the floor. Spread your legs and bend your knees, placing the soles of your feet together, and grasp your ankles with your hands. Your elbows should be resting on your knees. With your elbows, press your knees toward the floor as far down as they will go; hold the position for 10 seconds, and release. Be careful to avoid strain and pain. Do 12 times.

190. Sitting—forward stretch, legs straight, feet together

Sit on the floor with your legs straight out in front of you and your feet together. Holding your legs, slowly pull your torso forward and bring your head as close as possible to your knees without bending them. Hold the position for 12 seconds, and slowly sit straight again. Repeat 4 times.

101. On knees—lean back, thrust forward

Get down on your hands and knees, and stretch your straight arms out in front of you as far as you can, resting your buttocks on your heels. Hold the position for 10 seconds. Slowly push your torso forward, supporting yourself on straight arms and legs bent at the knees. Do not raise your shoulders. Hold the forward position for 10 seconds; then slowly return to the original position.

191. Prone—chest-lift

Lie prone with your legs stretched out, your arms bent at the elbows, and your palms on the floor under your shoulders. Turn your fingertips toward each other and raise your elbows slightly off the floor. Keeping your hipbones on the floor, slowly straighten up on your arms, pushing your chest and head off the floor as if doing a push-up. Hold your arms straight for 15 seconds, and slowly lower your chest to the floor. Repeat 4 times.

192. Kneeling—chest-stretch

Sit back, with your bottom on your heels and your knees bent. Shins and knees should be flat on the floor. Place your straight arms behind you, your palms on the floor. Slowly lift your bottom off your heels and push torso up as high as you can, arching your back. Hold the position for 15 seconds, and lower your bottom to your heels. Repeat 4 times.

193. Shoulder stand

Lie supine with your legs stretched out and your arms at your sides. Bend your knees; then slowly raise both legs into the air over your head. Resting your weight on your shoulders, bend your arms, keeping your upper triceps on the floor, but using your hands to support your body by holding your lower back. Slowly straighten your torso and legs; hold the position for 30 seconds, and slowly return to the original supine position.

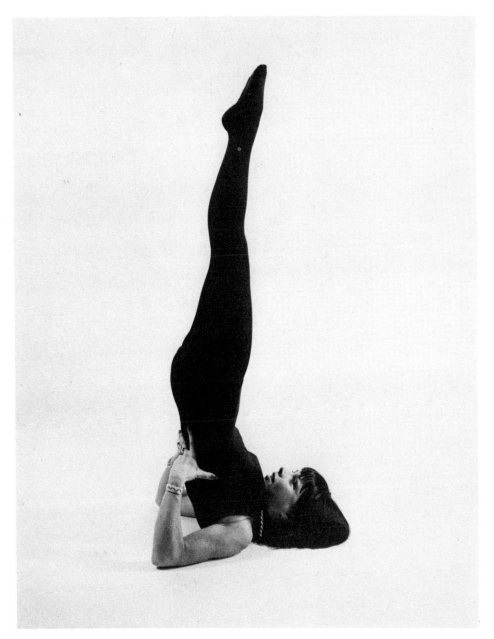

194. Standing—nose to knees

Stand with your feet together and your arms at your sides. Slowly bend forward and clasp the back of each calf with each hand. Keeping your legs *absolutely* straight, pull your torso toward your thighs and try to touch your nose to your knees. Go as far as you can without pain, and hold for 10 seconds. Then release and slowly stand straight again. Repeat 4 times.

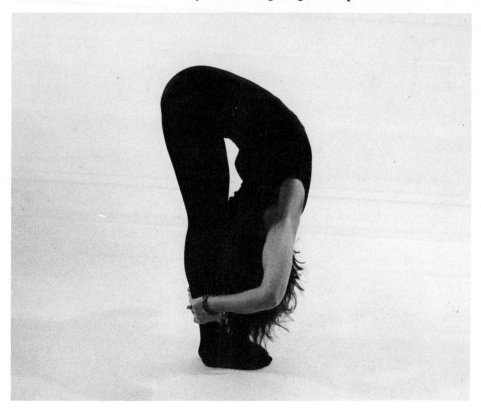

7

Pumping Iron; Lifting Bean Bags

Weight lifting does little, if anything, for your heart and circulation. In fact, under certain conditions, weight lifting can be dangerous, particularly to a beginner. If you have a heart condition and overexert yourself by lifting weights, you can do yourself serious damage. Never lift weights without your doctor's permission, especially if you suffer from lower-back pain and neck injuries.

As a rule, you should not lift weights after eating. The blood supply is concentrated in and around the digestive organs, and large quantities of fresh blood are needed to feed muscles straining to lift weights.

Neither in this book nor at Suzy Prudden Studios do we advocate weight lifting as an alternative form of physical fitness; instead, we have developed exercises which use moderate weights in a well-integrated physical fitness program designed to add shape, size, and tone to particular muscles of the human frame.

Most of the people who use weights in our fitness classes are women, who usually have underdeveloped muscle areas. We don't recommend weights for heavyset women; weights will only enlarge that which needs to be slimmed. But women with small breasts, skinny legs and arms, and flabby stomachs are encouraged to use three-pound weights in a series of easy exercises. They never go beyond five-pound weights, because the heavier the weight, the larger the muscle development. For most women, three pounds are usually sufficient.

If it is necessary for a man to use weights, we usually suggest a ten-to-fifteen pound limit. They are generally capable of working with heavier weights because they have larger masses of muscles. Many men, particularly those who have not exercised or played at sports since their college years, can firm up sagging muscles with the use of moderate weights, which are particularly useful in firming up paunchy stomachs and chests. Men who have lifted weights since their teen years and have always had well-developed muscles can use heavier weights. In fact, they have no choice if they want to keep their biceps and pectorals firm.

In addition to the small barbells and strap-on weights, we also provide two-pound bean bags for beginners which can be fastened on with connecting 145 straps and draped over ankles and wrists for particular exercises, all described at the end of this chapter. One such exercise, for men and women, begins with reclining on the elbows. The bean bags are draped over the ankles, and the student moves his legs in a bicycling motion. The exercise is not only superb for shaping up legs, but it flattens and firms stomachs as well.

These weights are practical for home use; they are easily stored and inexpensive to buy, an excellent investment in your body and self-esteem.

If you lift weights at home, first do our warm-ups. As with all other exercises, it is important to remember that a warm muscle is twenty percent more effective than a cold one. The alternative to warm-ups may be torn ligaments and excruciating pain. And both before and after lifting weights, do our stretchercises, so that muscles are not left in tensely contracted positions. Stretching before lifting weights will prevent an unsuspecting muscle from suddenly being wounded.

Don't overdo the lifting of weights; if you begin to feel aches and pains, stop; your muscles are telling you that you have done enough. And while exercising with weights, move slowly, careful not to pull a muscle in an unexpected direction. Your muscles will serve you well if you treat them with the care they deserve.

BUTTOCKS

195. Prone—weighted leg-lifts

Wrap a 3-pound ankle weight around each ankle and lie prone, resting your chin on folded arms. Keeping your hipbones on the floor, raise your right leg without bending the knee. Hold the leg in the air for 2 seconds; then lower it. Raise your left leg in the same manner. Repeat 16 times.

196. Weighted donkey-kick—knee-to-nose

With your 3-pound ankle weights strapped around your ankles, get down on your hands and knees, keeping your arms straight. Bring your right knee up under your body, trying to touch your nose. Bring your face down to meet your knee, and then kick your leg out behind you, raising it as high as you can while lifting your head. Repeat 6 times; then change legs.

UPPER BACK

66. On slant board, prone—weighted butterfly

Lie prone on a slant board, your head at the raised end, and stretch out your arms onto the floor, keeping them at right angles to your body. Grasp 3-pound weights in each hand and, still keeping your arms straight, raise and lower them like the wings of a butterfly. Repeat 8 times and rest.

BREASTS AND CHESTS

72. On slant board, supine—weighted butterfly

Lie supine on a slant board, your head at the raised end, your arms stretched out at right angles from your body and going to the floor. Grasp a 3-

pound weight in each hand and, keeping your arms straight, raise your hands off the floor to meet in the air above your chest. Slowly lower your arms and rest your hands on the floor again. Repeat 8 times.

197. On slant board, supine—weighted thresher

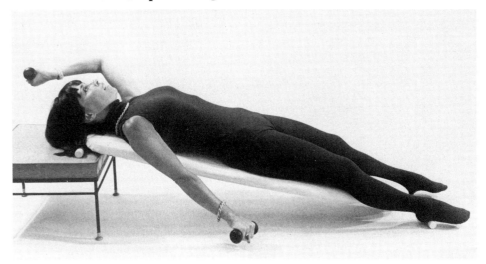

Lie supine on a slant board, your head at the raised end. Grasp 3-pound weights in each hand; then place your right arm at your side and stretch your left arm straight above your head. Alternate the straight-arm positions, and raise your straight right arm above your head, lowering your straight left arm to your side. Continue the alternation 16 times. If you prefer, this exercise can be done on the floor instead of on a slant board.

STOMACH

198. Sitting—weighted bent-knee leg-bounces

Place a 3-pound strap-on ankle weight around each ankle. Sit on the floor with your legs bent at the knees and your feet flat on the floor. Your legs should be slightly separated so that knees and feet are about 18 inches apart. Lean back on straight arms, resting your palms on the floor behind you. Raise your feet about 18 inches off the floor; then lower them to the floor again. Do 16 times in quick succession, and then relax.

STOMACH AND THIGHS

199. Weighted bicycle

With your 3-pound ankle weights strapped on, sit on the floor and lean back on your elbows and forearms. Raise your legs, moving them as if you were pedaling a bicycle. As you bring one leg up over your chest, your other leg should stretch straight out and at no time during the exercise should either of your legs touch the floor. Do this in a straight circular motion, repeating it 16 times.

147

200. Sitting in chair—weighted foot flex and half-point

Sit in a chair, cross your right leg over your left knee, and relax. Place a 3-pound strap-on weight around the ball and top of your foot. (Or take a 3-pound bean-bag weight and place it over the top of your foot near your toes.) Slowly flex your right foot, pulling your upper foot and toes up toward your body, and hold for 6 seconds. Then point only your foot, not your toes, downward, and hold for 6 seconds. (The weight will slide off if you point your toes.) Repeat 8 times; then change feet. Do 8 times with left foot, and repeat entire series once more.

CALVES AND ANKLES

201. Sitting in chair—weighted foot circle

Sit in a chair, cross your right leg over your left knee, and relax. Put a 3-pound strap-on weight around the ball and top of your foot. (Or put a 3-pound bean-bag weight over the top of your foot near your toes.) Keeping your toes flexed so that the weight doesn't slide off, slowly move your dangling right foot 8 times in a clockwise circular motion, then 8 times in a counter-clockwise motion. Repeat twice; then change legs. Switch again, and do the series twice only.

BACK, CHEST, AND BREASTS

202. Weighted paint the wall

Get down on your hands and knees and grasp a 3-pound weight in your right hand. As if you had a can of paint on your left side, and a paintbrush and a wall to paint on your right, reach with your right hand under your left side, and then swing your right hand back out and up toward the right, lifting it as high as you can. Do 4 times; then change arms. Grasp the 3-pound weight in your left hand, and repeat the exercise 4 times.

BACK, CHEST, AND ARMS

203. Weighted airplane stretch

Standing with your feet apart, grasp a 3-pound weight in each hand and bring your arms up to shoulder height. Bend them at the elbows until your knuckles touch in front of you; then slowly bring your elbows back as far as you can, and return them to the starting position, with your hands in front of you. Straighten your arms out to the sides, keeping them at shoulder height, and turn your fists upward. Return to original position, and repeat 12 times.

MIDRIFF AND ARMS

204. Weighted overhead arm-bounces

Stand with your feet apart, and grasp a 3-pound weight in each hand. Raise your left arm above your head and place your right hand beside your right knee. Arc your left hand over your head and bounce your torso to the right. Bounce 16 times; then reverse sides and bounce 16 times with your right arm arced over your head.

Posturing

Many people are formed into one posture or another: A posture can be the result of heredity, but it may also be the projection of inner emotion, a manifestation of a deep-seated self-image.

Poor posture is not just unattractive; it often results in severe back and neck pains, limiting one's physical pleasures. Beginning during the mid-twenties, the damaging effects of poor posture become more and more pronounced. By the late thirties, the stooper may find himself or herself periodically bedridden, suffering from debilitating backaches.

One of the most common posture problems is the "question mark" that rounds and hunches the backs of those who stand as if suffering from perpetual self-doubt. Another common problem is "dowager's hump." It occurs most often after the age of forty, the result of years of bad posture and little or no exercise. A more common problem is the abdominal (or abominable) "ski slope," a problem mainly associated with men but in these liberated times just as much a problem for women, too. This unattractive slope is caused by excess flab, weak abdominals, and strained lower-back muscles.

Our posturecises are easy to do and can correct many particular posture problems. Thereafter, you can concentrate on your overall fitness. But the longer you wait, the more difficult it becomes to correct a chronic problem.

Many people become habituated to bad posture, though good posture is just as habit-forming and far more comfortable. Our posture exercises will straighten you out, but don't expect to achieve major results overnight. Improvement will be progressive, occurring little by little. If you have a serious posture problem, particularly scoliosis (a lateral curvature of the spine), check with your doctor before beginning our posturecises.

Basic Posture Problems

ROUND SHOULDERS

5. Corner push-ups

At a distance of about 2 to 3 feet face a corner of a room and stand with your feet together. Place your palms against each wall of the corner, your arms at shoulder height. Keeping your body straight, lean forward, bringing your face and chest as close to the corner as possible; then push off, back to an erect position. Repeat 8 times, keeping your elbows at shoulder height at all times.

183. Push-ups

Assume a push-up position, supporting yourself on your palms and the balls of your feet. Keeping your body straight, slowly lower yourself, letting your chest touch the floor first. Once down, relax. Get up any way you feel comfortable, and assume the push-up position again. As you lower yourself,

149

(cont'd)

count to 6 and do 4 times. When you're strong enough you'll be able to raise your straight body in the push-up position.

19. Airplane stretch

Standing with your feet apart, bring your arms up to shoulder height. Bend them at the elbows until your fingers touch in front of you, and then quickly bring your elbows back as far as you can, and return them to the starting position with your hands in front of you. Straighten your arms out to the sides, keeping them at shoulder height, and turn your palms upward. Return to the original position, and repeat 12 times.

18. The back of my hand

This exercise can be done with feet either together or apart. Keep your left arm at your side and raise your right, bending it at the elbow. Place the back of your right hand against your right cheek, and swing your arm, stretching your hand back and away from your face until your arm is as straight as a backstroker's. Do the same with your left hand and arm, keeping your right at your side. Do each arm 8 times.

112. Body stretch

This can be done standing, sitting, or lying down.

A. Standing: Stretch your arms above your head, stand on your toes, and stretch your body as hard as you can. Hold the stretched position for 4 seconds and relax. Repeat 4 times.

B. Sitting: Sit with your feet flat on the floor and your knees bent. Raise your arms straight up, clasping your hands above your head, and stretch as hard as you can. Hold the stretched position for 4 seconds and relax. Repeat 4 times.

C. Lying. Lie prone or supine, stretching your arms on the floor straight above your head. Point your toes and stretch your body, legs, and arms as hard as you can. Hold the stretched position for 4 seconds and then relax. Repeat 4 times.

4. Prone—arm-lifts

Lie prone with your chin on the floor and your arms stretched out straight in front of you. Lift your right arm into the air as high as you can, keeping it beside your ear and keeping your chin on the floor. Lower your right arm; then lift the left arm in the same manner. Repeat 16 times.

64. Prone—double arm-lifts

Lie prone with your chin on the floor and your arms stretched out straight on the floor above your head. Anchor your feet under something secure. Raise both straight arms, your head, and your chest off the floor as high as you can. Hold the position for 4 seconds; then return to your original position for 4 more seconds. Repeat 8 times.

85. Airplane stretch and circle

Stand with your feet apart, fingertips of both hands touching in front of your chest, elbows out at your sides at shoulder height. Gently bring your elbows back behind you as far as they can go; then touch fingertips again.

Straighten your arms out in front of you, raise them straight up, then back, and then down, making a full circular motion. Return to the original position, and repeat entire exercise 8 times. Then reverse circular motion and repeat 8 times.

65. Pushing marbles with your nose

Get down on your hands and knees and stretch your arms out as far as you can in front of you while resting your bottom on your heels. Move your torso forward, keeping your head close to the floor as if pushing an imaginary marble with your nose. Your head will pass your arms, which will be bent at the elbows. After your nose has gone as far as possible, raise your head, straightening your arms, and push your entire torso upward. Return to the original position with your bottom on your heels, and repeat the exercise 4 times.

75. Dowel—shoulder rotate

Hold a 3-foot dowel at each end in front of your thighs, keeping your arms straight. Slowly raise your straight arms up in front of you and above your head; then continue moving your arms back as far as you can, always keeping those arms straight. When your arms have reached as far back as they can go without pain, bend them at the elbows and lower them until the dowel is just behind your buttocks and your arms are straight again. Slowly raise your straight arms up behind you as far as you can. When your arms have reached as far up as they can go without pain, bend them at the elbows and continue raising them until they stretch straight up over your head. Slowly lower your straight arms in front of you until the dowel is against your upper thighs. Do 16 times.

SWAYBACK

27. Back—arch and flatten

Lie supine, bend your knees to a 90-degree angle, and keep your feet flat on the floor. With your upper back and bottom on the floor, gently arch your lower back. Then flatten it, gently pressing it against the floor. Hold the flattened position for 4 seconds, and repeat the entire exercise 6 times.

1. Back flat—leg-lower

This exercise is essential for lower-back strength. If you feel pain in your lower back, make sure you are doing it correctly. This exercise often seems to require more effort than it's worth, but, although slow in showing progress, it's one of the most important.

Lie supine. Bring your knees over your chest and then straighten your legs so that they form a 90-degree angle with your torso and the floor. Keeping the small of your back pressed firmly against the floor, slowly lower your legs *only* as far as you can without your back rising off the floor. (If you feel your back rising, you have lowered your legs too far.) At that point, hold the position for 4 seconds; then release by bending your knees over your chest. Rest and repeat 4 times. *Never* lower your legs all the way down to the floor; that will cause back strain. For illustration, see page 15.

176. Supine—hip-lift

Lie supine. Bend your knees with your feet flat on the floor, and rest your arms at your sides, your palms on the floor. Lift your buttocks off the floor, pushing your hips up toward the ceiling. Hold the position for 4 seconds; then slowly lower your buttocks to the floor again. Repeat 6 times.

61. The metronome

Lie supine. Raise your legs, bending your knees over your chest. Press the small of your back against the floor and slowly lower your bent legs to the left, trying to keep both shoulders on the floor. Lift your bent legs off the floor, bringing them over your chest again and pressing the small of your back against the floor. Slowly lower your legs to the right. Repeat 16 times.

63. The feline

Get down on your hands and knees. Slowly lower your head and round your back, lifting it up while you suck in your stomach. Hold the position for 3 seconds, then raise your head up and slowly lower your back, letting it sag in the middle. Repeat 8 times.

22. Bent-knee sit-ups

Sit on the floor with your knees bent, and anchor your feet under a couch, dresser, or piece of sturdy furniture. Clasp your hands behind your neck and from this sitting position slowly lie down. When your back is flat on the floor, sit up, keeping your hands clasped behind your neck. Be sure to come up with a rounded, not a straight, back, straighten your back only when you have reached the final sitting position. Start with 5, and work up to whatever is comfortable.

23. Bicycle

Sit on the floor and lean back on your elbows and forearms. Raise your legs, moving them as if you were pedaling a bicycle; as you bring one leg up over your chest, your other leg should stretch straight out. At no time during the exercise should your legs touch the floor. Maintaining a straight circular motion, repeat 16 times.

173. On table—leg-lifts

Place your torso in a prone position across a low table or bench, and let your legs hang down to the floor. Holding onto the table or bench, lift both your legs into the air and straighten them out behind you. Lift them as high as you can, hold them up for 4 seconds, then relax them to the floor. Do 6 times.

185. Leg-to-chest back-press

Lie supine with your legs stretched out, your arms at your sides, and the back of your head on the floor. Raise your head, looking down toward your stomach, and lift your right leg, bending it at the knee and raising it over your chest. Clasp your hands around your right shin, just under the knee, and pull your right leg against your chest, as you press your lower back against the
floor. Hold the position for 4 seconds; then alternate legs. Repeat 8 times.

Check with your doctor before doing exercises for a scoliosis.

205. Lie on a book—arm raises

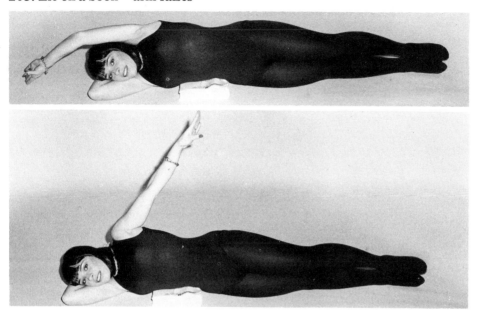

If your back curves to the right (i.e., a backward C), lie on your right side, placing a book just under your rib cage. Rest your head on your folded right arm, and lay your left arm on your left side. Keeping your body and your left arm straight, raise your left arm up, stretching your left hand over your head. Hold the position for 4 seconds; then return your straight left arm to your side. Repeat 6 times. If your back curves to the left, do the exercise on your left side.

206. Side-to-side bounce, arm over head

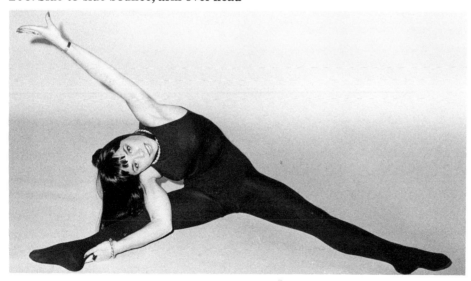

Sit with your legs moderately wide apart and stretched out straight. If your back curves to the right, place your right hand, palm up, under your 153

(cont'd)

right calf. Raise your left arm and curve it over your head. Bounce your torso to the side, trying to touch your right ear to your right knee, without bending the knee. Repeat 12 times. Change sides and put both hands on your left knee; bounce your torso forward and back, trying to touch your nose to your left knee without bending the knee. Repeat 12 times. If your back curves to the left, do the exercise bouncing on your left side with your right arm arcing above your head, and to your right side holding your knee with both hands.

Feet

DUCK FEET

207. Walk pigeon-toed

Turn your toes inward and walk around the room like a pigeon.

PIGEON TOES

208. Walk like a duck

Turn your feet out and walk around the room like a duck.

FLAT FEET

209. Walk on the outside

Lean on the outsides of your feet and walk around the room. (This exercise is good for knock-knees, too.)

CURVED ANKLES (OUTWARD)

210. Walk on the inside

Lean on the insides of your feet and walk around the room. (This exercise is good for bowlegs, too.)

FOR HEALTHY FEET

211. Walk

Put on a pair of comfortable, sturdy shoes and just walk.

36. Heel-up

Stand with your feet together and your hands at your sides. Raise your right heel by going up on the ball and toes of your right foot, leaning your weight on your left leg. Alternate from right leg to left leg, holding each position to a count of 3. Repeat alternation 16 times.

37. Toe flex and curl

Stand with your feet together and curl your toes under as if trying to pick up a pencil with them. Hold the position for 2 seconds. Uncurl your toes and pull them up toward your body. Hold that position for 2 seconds. Repeat 8 times.

39. Curl feet and flatten

Stand with your feet together and your arms at your sides. Shift so that your weight is on the outsides of your feet, and curl your toes under. Hold the position for 4 seconds; then return to a flat-footed stance. Do 8 times.

40. Toe stretch and release

This exercise may be done while standing, sitting, or even lying down, but be sure your feet are bare. Stretch and separate your toes, holding this position for 4 seconds, before releasing your muscles. Repeat 10 times with each foot. Then curl your toes under and hold that position for 2 seconds to release the tension in your foot. If your foot cramps, do the exercise 4 times only, and don't continue while your foot is cramped. You can do it later.

8

Cellulite: Every Body's Problem

In recent years, cellulite has received considerable publicity, especially as a problem which afflicts women. What is not so widely known is that cellulite also afflicts men and teen-agers of both sexes.

Cellulite is a condition which puckers the outer layers of the skin on thighs, hips, and bottoms, making the skin resemble oatmeal.

All of the affected areas, whether soft or hard, can be made to experience pain simply by squeezing them. And the pain is often out of proportion to the pressure exerted. The pain is the result of too much fiber being compressed into too small an area.

Cellulite has been recognized as a problem, and it has become almost chic to receive "cellulite treatments." We deal with this condition not because it is trendy, but because it is a disfiguring problem which diminishes health and self-esteem.

Walk along any beach during the summer and you will observe that cellulite is a common problem. Though most sufferers are aware only of the aesthetic misfortune of cellulite, health problems come into play, too. Cellulite is often accompanied by high levels of cholesterol which can lead to arteriosclerosis.

What causes cellulite? Three components, working in insidious concert: tension, fatty foods in abundance, and insufficient exercise.

In woman, the condition commonly manifests itself on hips, thighs, and buttocks. And a considerable proportion of the male and female population have cellulite across their abdomens and lower backs, hardly contributing to trim figures. But there is hope; cellulite can be diminished and in many cases entirely eliminated.

The first step in the therapy is awareness of the problem. Face your moment of truth by standing naked in front of a full-length mirror and decide what improvements you want to make.

Cellulite responds remarkably well to a three-pronged attack of exercise, massage, and diet. Massage is useful until the condition has been eliminated; afterwards, sensible diet and proper exercise will keep your body trim and attractive. If you have cellulite, massage helps to break up soft congested fat cells.

At first meetings of all cellulite workshops, we warn students that no matter how much they massage and exercise, they will not achieve satisfactory results with a diet that includes alcohol, sugar, cheese, fatty meats, cream, most snack foods, etc.

We also point out an additional and interesting factor: Doctors have documented that fat cells are often inherited. If you have one fat parent, you have a better than fifty percent chance of being fat, too. If both your parents are fat, the odds rise to seventy-five percent. Obese parents often have compulsive eating habits. As models, they pass on those habits to their children. Excess weight is closely related to cellulite, so the overall problem of obesity must be treated while applying treatment to particular areas of the body.

There are also many thin people afflicted with unsightly cellulite; they, too, can reshape themselves.

Cellulite develops insidiously. From day to day you hardly notice any change in your body; six to ten months later, the condition is depressingly apparent. But it doesn't take that long to eliminate; improvement can be seen within ten days, and if you are really conscientious, you can expect surprisingly positive results within a month.

We knew a woman, a well-known actress, who gained too much weight during her pregnancy; after the baby was born, she went on an eating spree. Within a year, her body became disfigured—flabby, and marred by cellulite. Luckily, she woke up in time. Eliminating alcohol and fatty foods from her diet, she also exercised at our studios and learned to massage the affected areas. Today, she is as lovely and feminine as she had ever been, and her skin is tight over long, elegant muscles. If anything, her look is one of athletic chic.

Exercise it Away

Areas affected by cellulite should be exercised daily for fifteen to thirty minutes, depending on your endurance, health, and determination to improve.

Exercise not only burns up calories, it diminishes the bulky presence of cellulite. In addition to toning muscles, exercise converts one pound of fat to five pounds of muscle. At the end of this chapter are the exercises we have found to be most effective in reducing cellulite.

Eat It Away

We have already mentioned various foods which contribute to the development of cellulite. Now here are foods you can eat freely: salads (without rich cheesy dressings); fruits and vegetables (especially raw and unprocessed); nonfat milk and its by-products; poultry (except for duck); fish (except for shellfish, which contain inordinately high amounts of cholesterol); wheat germ; yogurt in moderation; cottage cheese; gelatin; natural, unsweetened fruit juices; and especially water. Water is an indispensable aid to elimination, cleansing the body of waste materials. To flush out your digestive system, we recommend you drink about forty-eight ounces of water a day. Such a quantity will aid digestion, and at the same time decrease the chances of developing cellulite. However, one should spread those forty-eight ounces out over fourteen to sixteen hours.

Salt is a highly controversial substance. While it is necessary for human life, for medical reasons many diets must be relatively free of salt. In addition, a diet rich in salt will cause superfluous water retention that can add to cellulite. We suggest you consult your doctor about the desirable amount of salt in your diet.

Massage It Away

While exercise converts fat to muscle, massage breaks up pockets of cellulite.

During a recent cellulite workshop at Suzy Prudden Studios, one woman lost an inch of cellulite on each of her thighs after only two weeks of intensive, cellulite massage. The actual massage begins gently, accustoming the flesh to a pulling-pushing movement. Then the flesh is gently, but firmly, kneaded as if kneading baker's dough. Throughout the process, care is taken not to pinch or bruise delicate areas. Next, portions of the flesh are gently twisted back and forth as if making a figure S, then reversed to a figure Z, without applying too much pressure. Finally, a large section of cellulite is grasped and wrung out like a wet towel.

During massage, never rub the insides or the lower backs of the thighs, those areas are thick with veins and capillaries which can be easily bruised or otherwise damaged.

Though tension massage should be administered by professionals, we recommend that each of you learn to do your own cellulite massage. It's the only way to avoid the pain that comes from the application of too much pressure.

Once cellulite has been eliminated, you need only a regular fitness program and a sensible diet. As you should never overdo exercise, you should not overdo massage either, and always be careful to avoid areas where veins and capillaries are near the surface of the skin.

At home, we suggest warm showers or baths as appropriate environments in which to administer massage. There the muscles are warm and malleable, and massage can prove highly effective.

UPPER ARMS

11. Shoulder twist

Stand with your feet slightly apart and your arms out to your sides at shoulder height. Stretching your arms outward, turn your palms up. Then slowly turn your palms forward, down, and up behind, allowing your shoulders to rotate forward. Hold the position 4 seconds, and return to forward palms-up position for 4 seconds. Repeat 8 times.

CELLULITE: EVERY BODY'S PROBLEM

18. The back of my hand

This exercise can be done with feet together or apart. Keep your left arm at your side, and raise your right arm, bending it at the elbow. Place the back of your right hand against your right cheek. Then swing your arm, stretching your hand back and away from your face until your arm is as straight as a backstroker's. Do the same with your left hand and arm, with your right at your side. Do each arm 8 times.

73. Shoulder rotate

Stand with your feet apart and your arms raised at your sides to shoulder height. Turn your right hand and arm under, turning your right shoulder forward; at the same time, turn your left hand and arm backward, turning your left shoulder back. Change direction of both arms, turning left hand down and right hand up. Repeat 12 times.

MIDRIFF

89. Arm-swing

Stand with your feet apart and your arms stretched out to the sides level with your shoulders. Swing both arms, first to the left, then to the right, following the movement with your nose. Throughout, keep your hips from moving. Do 16 times.

135. Washing machine

Stand with your feet apart and bend forward from the hips, your body making a right angle. Bend your arms at the elbows, so that they form right angles, too. Twist your body up and down from the waist, moving your torso and arms like the agitating motion of a washing machine. Repeat 16 times.

LOVE HANDLES

58. Holding hands—side-to-side bounce

Stand with your feet apart and stretch your arms up, clasping your hands together above your head. From your waist, arc your body to the right, without turning your body to the side. Bounce your torso 4 times over your right leg. Change direction, arcing your body to the left, and bounce 4 more times. Be sure to stretch your arms as you bounce.

60. Elbow snap

Standing with your legs apart, hold your arms at shoulder height and bend them at the elbows. Turn your torso twice to the right, twice to the left. While twisting your torso, keep your legs stationary and don't move your hips. Twist 16 times in each direction.

BOTTOM

7. Donkey-kick—knee-to-nose

Get down on your hands and knees, keeping your arms straight. Bring your right knee up under your body, trying to touch your nose, and bring 159 your face down to meet your knee. Kick your leg out behind you, raising it as high as you can while lifting your head. Repeat 6 times, then change legs.

28. Prone—tighten and release

Lie in a prone position, resting your forehead or your chin on folded arms. Tighten your abdominals, buttock muscles, inner thighs, and vaginal muscles. Hold all contractions for 4 seconds, then release. Repeat 6 times.

THIGHS

34. On elbow—leg-lift

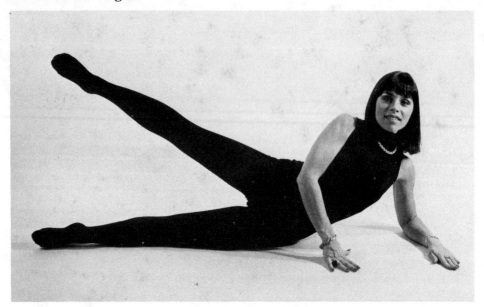

Lie on one side of your body; then raise your torso off the floor by propping yourself on an elbow, using forearm and hip for support. Lift your upper leg, like half a scissors, up and down 6 times. Keep your toes pointed, then repeat 6 times with flexed feet, being sure to keep your torso straight. Change sides and repeat.

35. On side—under leg-lift

Lie on your right side, resting your head on your right bicep to cushion your head from the floor. Bend your left leg, placing your left foot behind your right knee. Lift your right leg as far as you can, then lower it. Do 6 times with toes pointed and 6 times with foot flexed, then switch sides and repeat, raising left foot and bending right leg.

48. On elbows—scissors crossover

Sit on the floor, leaning back on your elbows and forearms. Keeping your legs apart, lift them off the floor with your feet flexed and turned outward. Then turn your feet inward, keeping your legs straight, and cross your feet in front of you, right leg over left leg. From the crossed position, turn your feet outward, and return legs to the spread position, keeping your feet and legs off the floor. Turn your feet inward again and cross them in front of you, this time left leg over right leg. From the crossed position, turn your feet outward and return to spread-legs position. Repeat 8 times. (If this gives you lower-back pain, wait a few minutes before trying it again.)

212. On side—scissors

Lean over on your right side, resting on your right elbow and forearm; put your left hand behind you to balance yourself. Raise both straight legs. Repeat scissors motion, lifting your right leg into the air as left leg is lowered close to the floor and is then crossed over the right. Do 8 times, then lean on your left side, resting on your left elbow and forearm with your right hand behind you to balance yourself. Raise both straight legs. Repeat the scissors motion, lifting your left leg into the air as you lower your right leg close to the floor and then cross it over your left leg. Repeat 8 times.

49. Infinity leg-swing

Sit on the floor, lean back on your elbows and forearms, and stretch your legs out in front of you. Flex your right foot and lift it, turning it to the left. Cross it over your left leg until you can place your right big toe just beyond your left leg. Reverse the motion, bringing your right foot back wide and turning the entire foot to the right. Repeat 8 times and change legs.

50. Sitting, L position—leg-lifts

Sit on the floor with your left leg bent at the knee, your left calf crossing in front of your crotch and your left foot pointed toward your right leg. Bend your right leg at your side, your right calf beside, but not touching, your right buttock, and your right foot pointing behind you. Rest your palms on the floor behind you, but don't place your weight on them; they are there for balance only. Keeping your body straight and your right leg bent, raise and lower your right leg 12 times. Reverse the position of your legs, crossing your right leg in front of you and bending your left leg to your left side. Raise and lower your left leg 12 times. Repeat series twice.

51. Sitting, L position—leg-lift and stretch

Sit as in the above exercise, with your left leg bent and crossed in front of you and your right leg bent out to your right side. Keep your body facing forward and rest on your palms placed behind you. Raise your right leg, keeping it out to the side, and when the entire leg is 3 to 6 inches off the floor, straighten it out to the side. Hold the position for 3 seconds, return to a bent-knee position, and lower your leg to the floor. Repeat 6 times. Be sure to hold your torso upright, and don't lean your weight on your hands. Reverse the position, crossing your right leg in front of you and bending your left leg out to the side, and repeat exercise 6 times with your left leg. Do series twice.

9

Food for Thought—
Thoughts on Nutrition

There is hardly an adult in the western world who is not to some extent aware of the importance of nutrition. It has been positioned as one of the greatest popular sciences of the day, and the public's interest is nothing less than a proper concern for their own health, fitness, longevity, and general well-being.

Despite heavy advertising and publicity, proper nutrition is unknown to many. In this chapter, we hope to fill the gaps and provide some solid information to improve the quality of your diet.

You Are My Sugar

Sugar contains relatively high amounts of calories, but calories that have been robbed of vitamins, minerals, and even vital amino acids. When people get insufficient supplies of protein and natural (unrefined) sugar from fresh sources of carbohydrates (uncooked fruits and vegetables), they may develop an appetite, as well as a need for, refined sugar.

Some medical authorities think that an overconsumption of refined sugar causes sugar levels to go up and down like waves on a graph. During periods when blood sugar is especially low, the pancreas is stimulated to react, producing excess insulin.

The alternative is quite simple: If you consume sugar from fruits and vegetables, your blood-sugar level will adjust itself, and you will not be troubled by the swings of an emotional pendulum. If you are concerned about your blood-sugar levels, see an endocrinologist; such a doctor can administer a painless test to determine the levels of blood sugar.

If you don't want to eliminate refined sugars from your diet, we suggest they play a minimal role in your daily nutrition. For instance, have a dessert after dinner, but avoid refined sugars throughout the rest of the day. If a craving for something sweet overcomes you, then have a piece of sweet fresh fruit.

Caffeined

Caffeine, so often used to excess, is an alkaloid found most commonly in coffee, cola drinks, and, to a lesser degree, in tea. Most Americans and Europeans start each day with a cup of coffee that contains about 100 milligrams of caffeine, a potent stimulant to the central nervous system. Unfortunately, many people don't stop with the first 100 milligrams; they may consume up to 1,000 milligrams of caffeine daily. The result is an inordinately increased heartbeat and pulse rate and a general nervousness. Consequently, the amount of plasma pumped through the kidneys is significantly increased. Heart-attack victims are frequently advised to eliminate caffeine from their diets, as are those who suffer from high blood pressure.

Nutritionists have pointed out that excessive intake of caffeine can actually lead to vitamin B deficiencies. Vitamin B loss takes place because caffeine is a diuretic, and the essential vitamin is passed out in the urine. In addition, it is widely known that caffeine can, and often does, result in insomnia. Those who rely on sleeping pills every night will also require several strong cups of coffee in the morning. In time, of course, the doses must be increased; thus the state of one's health is decreased.

The expression "coffee break" is ironic. Those who request a fifteen-minute interval from work as a time in which to relax and enjoy a calming cup of coffee are really only heightening their tension. Coffee, a high-acid liquid, only aggravates any tensions that may be present. Those already suffering from ulcers are warned not to drink coffee, tea, or cola drinks.

Caffeine can also have an adverse effect on blood sugar. A single cup of coffee may stimulate the liver, in effect forcing sugar out of the liver. The initial result is a surge of energy—that quickly dwindles away. Comparative fatigue results after the secreted sugar has been quickly dissipated. With the sugar level reduced, the body compensates with a craving for something sweet. Hypoglycemia may be a not too distant result, and it can be caused by refined sugars, caffeine, and alcohol, the last affects the liver similarly to the way it is affected by caffeine.

If you misuse alcohol, sugar, or caffeine, you will experience highs and lows throughout each day. At first, they may be energy levels only; but in time, they will become emotional peaks and valleys.

Pillars of Salt

Salt plays a more ambiguous role in human nutrition. Common table salt is eliminated from the diets of those with heart conditions; yet salt itself can never be eliminated from the human body, nor should it be, since it is essential for life itself.

However, excessive salt intake may cause retention of water in the body and cause blood pressure to rise in predisposed individuals.

If you have a tendency to retain water, or if you think you have high blood pressure, discuss these problems with a nutritionist who will regulate the amounts of salt and diuretics appropriate for you.

163

As one grows into one's thirties and forties, many nutritionists believe that one's levels of water retention significantly increases. Therefore, people are advised to cut down on salt intake, especially since heart attacks increase markedly during that age span. A salt-restricted diet benefits those suffering from hypertension as well.

The Three Best

Proteins, carbohydrates, and fats are absolutely essential for life. Without adequate supplies of any of the three, you will be malnourished.

Let's begin with the most misunderstood of the substances: fats. If taken in excess, fats can aggravate the development of arteriosclerosis in predisposed individuals. However, taken in moderation, fat is an excellent nutrient. In order to judge the value of fat, you should know that a single gram of fat yields nine calories, and that no more than thirty percent of your diet should consist of fat. If fat was not present, the four essential vitamins (A, D, E, and K) could not be properly absorbed, for they are fat soluble.

There are fats, and there are fats. The good fats are polyunsaturated, the bad ones saturated. Excessive intake of saturated fats can lead to hyper-cholesterolemia, or high blood cholesterol in certain individuals. Common sources of saturated fats are fatty beef, eggs, and butter. While saturated fats can be manufactured by the body from other food substances, polyunsaturated fats must be eaten because the body cannot manufacture them. You have only to read the labels of cooking oils and margarines in order to discover which are made from polyunsaturated fats. The most desirable fatty acids exist in abundant supply in corn oil, safflower oil, and soybean oil, all of which are used to make margarines.

Proteins are the building blocks of life, vital to muscle development as well as to a variety of body tissues. Protein is less caloric than fat; one gram yields a mere four calories. In a well-balanced diet, protein should comprise not less than fourteen percent of the diet's nutritional value. Nutritionists and doctors suggest that most people consume at least two and a half to three ounces of protein a day, about seventy grams. Primary sources of protein are fish, poultry, lean beef, cheese, milk, eggs, nuts, and soybeans. Their regular consumption ensures the vital rebirth of essential cells and the maintenance of cells in a healthy condition; at the same time, they provide the body with energy.

Protein is composed of carbon, hydrogen, nitrogen, and oxygen, all linked in chains of amino-acid molecules. During the metabolic process of digestion, proteins are broken down so they may do their work effectively. Once they reach the small intestine, amino acids are released and subsequently move through the blood, heading for different cells where damaged areas are repaired and new cells are born.

There are two kinds of amino acids—essential and nonessential. Essential amino acids, required by the human body, cannot be synthesized by the digestive system and can be obtained only from the inclusion in the daily diet of proteins. Nonessential amino acids are synthesized by the digestive system, and, when the body requires them, the digestive system positively responds.

Carbohydrates, obtained from fresh fruits and vegetables, are sources of the most enduring energy. Refined, granulated sugar comes from sugar cane, the sugar beet, or sorghum. Junk foods, rich in refined sugars, are full of superfluous calories, usually between 200 and 250. However, one delicious peach has only thirty-five calories. One gram of carbohydrates yields a mere four calories.

Unfortunately, most people consume too many low-quality carbohydrates, which can easily lead to unhealthful deposits of fat within the body. Many nutritionists are concerned that millions of Americans are getting by on an overabundance of low-quality carbohydrates, which can only reduce health and longevity.

Vital Vitamins

If everyone ate three well-balanced meals a day, few people would require additional vitamins, for their diets would contain an adequate supply. In fact, if you read the labels on most vitamin bottles, you will notice that consumption of vitamins is regarded as supplementary. In other words, you should get all the necessary vitamins from your daily diet, but if you don't eat well-balanced meals, you should certainly take vitamin supplements.

Cumulative vitamin deficiencies often result in a wide assortment of maladies, but they can be countered with adequate vitamin supplements. On the other hand, certain vitamins, if taken excessively, can be dangerous, for they have a toxicity level.

All vitamins can be separated into two categories: Those which are soluble in water (B-complex and C) and those which are soluble in fat (vitamins A, D, E, and K). Those which are fat-soluble can be stored in the body; those which are water-soluble must be taken every day, for they are eliminated from the body in urine.

From the Top: A

Vitamin A is abundant in carrots, beets, milk, tomatoes, liver, and fish-liver oils. Vegetables as a source of vitamin A should be fresh and uncooked.

Though its benefits are manifold, vitamin A's best-known virtue is as an aid in the prevention of night blindness. It is less well-known that it helps to maintain a youthful skin texture and assists the proper functioning of mucus membranes. Nutritionists have suggested that each adult needs between 5,000 and 10,000 international units of vitamin A each day. However, that does not seem to allow for accumulations of this fat-soluble substance. And large quantities of vitamin A can cause damage; therefore, the Food and Drug Administration has stated that any preparation of vitamin A containing more than 10,000 international units cannot be dispensed without a prescription. Nutritionists believe that toxicity from vitamin A will result only after massive daily doses (100,000 i.u.) taken over a period of several months.

We believe that common sense dictates that you consult your physician before taking a vitamin A supplement.

B is Complex

The B complex of vitamins comprise an entire division within the army of vitamins; their effects are manifold, and their importance should not be underestimated. The very presence or absence of one ingredient affects all the others in the B complex. If your body lacks one of the B vitamins, you will have a deficiency of all the others as well. Similarly, if you increase the amounts of any one B vitamin, you will have to increase all of the B vitamins. And since they are water-soluble, they are not stored in the body and must be replaced daily.

Many nutritionists advise a vitamin B complex to be taken as a supplement even if one consumes three well-balanced meals a day; they believe that millions of Americans suffer from mild forms of B vitamin deficiencies because of food preparation and processing methods. B vitamins are destroyed either by cooking or canning, and refined grains have been stripped of their essential vitamins.

The complex is composed of B-1, B-2, B-6, and B-12; there are no such B vitamins as B-3, B-4, B-5, B-7, B-8, B-9, B-10, or B-11. Such designations have been dropped, for they had been erroneously applied in the first place.

B-1, also known as thiamine, is essential for carbohydrate metabolism, as well as for the regular elimination of waste materials. It also contributes to growth. As a co-enzyme, it is particularly well utilized to convert glucose into energy, helping to bring oxygen to various parts of the body. The recommended daily allowance is .4 milligrams. Recently, B-1 has been advertised as a substance helpful in combating the effects of stress and tension. Without B-1, you might suffer from fatigue, constipation, flatulence, and nervousness. In extreme cases, a deficiency may cause enlargement of the heart and even beriberi.

The natural sources are wheat germ, whole grains, yeast, eggs, soybeans, nuts, liver, and milk.

Vitamin B-2, also known as riboflavin, helps to maintain the healthy glow of the skin. Even more important, it protects the cornea of the eye and contributes to the healthy functioning of the nervous system while improving the oxidation of cells and tissues. The most obvious signs of vitamin B-2 deficiency are cracks in the skin, especially around the orifices of the body.

The best natural sources of B-2 are fresh, leafy greens, wheat germ, milk, liver, yeast, and eggs.

Vitamin B-6, also known as pyridoxine, helps the body to utilize fats and proteins, to build healthy blood cells. In addition, B-6 contributes to the proper functioning of the nervous system, especially the brain. For years, B-6 has been employed to treat an unusual form of anemia.

Natural sources are wheat germ, eggs, yeast, liver, kidney, and milk.

Vitamin B-12, also known as cyanocobalamin, has been effectively used
in treating various types of anemia, too. It is essential to the formation of

strong red-blood cells, for it goes right to the marrow of the bones. A lack of B-12 can lead to pernicious anemia.

The single best source of B-12 is liver; other sources include kidneys, brains, eggs, milk, and cheese.

Included in the B complex are other substances not given either letters or numbers. They are inositol, niacin, biotin, folic acid, pantothenic acid, choline, and para-aminobenzoic acid.

Inositol helps the body to absorb vitamin E and to diminish levels of cholesterol, for it is structurally related to lecithin, another important enemy of cholesterol.

Though a precise need, in humans, for inositol has not been satisfactorily established, a deficiency causes various deleterious effects in laboratory animals, such as eczema and baldness. In addition to a vitamin B-complex pill, inositol can be obtained from liver, kidney, wheat germ, soybean, and whole grain.

Niacin has long been highly regarded as a positive influence on the central nervous system and the healthy functioning of the liver. As a co-enzyme, it acts in the oxidation of carbohydrates, particularly starches and sugars. Massive doses will lower cholesterol in the bloodstream, but you must discuss the specific dosage with your doctor.

A niacin deficiency can cause serious problems, the worst being pellagra. In addition, many emotional conditions, such as mild paranoia and hostility, have been traced to niacin deficiencies.

Niacin is found in fish, liver, kidney, leafy greens, yeast, and wheat germ. The body also manufactures an amino acid, tryptophan, which can be converted into niacin.

Biotin was once known as vitamin H; it assists in the digestion of fats. Nutritionists and researchers have done comparatively little work on biotin; but it has been proven that the body creates it in the intestines. Other sources include wheat germ, liver, and yeast.

Folic acid is another co-enzyme which helps the body to properly use an assortment of amino acids and sugar. Some nutritionists believe that folic acid can help to prevent baldness; as far as we know, that has not yet been proven in controlled, laboratory conditions.

According to the Food and Drug Administration, more than .1 milligram of folic acid cannot be sold over the counter without a prescription, for it may conceal the symptoms of anemia. Apparently folic acid contributes to the development of red-blood cells, and its presence can interfere with the diagnosis of anemia.

In addition to most vitamin B-complex preparations, you can find folic acid in yeast, liver, kidney, and leafy greens.

Pantothenic acid is important to the overall digestive process, but it is particularly important to carbohydrate metabolism. It, too, plays a significant role in the health of various adrenal glands.

Sufferers from stress may burn up great quantities of pantothenic acid, which is why the entire B-complex is now being marketed to those especially susceptible to the effects of intense stress and tension.

167

Meat, yeast, soybeans, and peas contain pantothenic acid; if necessary, your doctor can prescribe a supplementary dosage.

Choline plays an influential role in reducing cholesterol levels as well as high-blood pressure. Though the body manufactures choline, you can find generous supplies in yeast, wheat germ, liver, kidney, and leafy greens.

Last among the elements of the B-complex is para-aminobenzoic acid, also known as P.A.B.A., and it is closely related to folic acid. P.A.B.A. is a potent substance; thirty milligrams or more will render sulphur drugs ineffectual. Therefore, the F.D.A. prevents consumers from buying more than thirty milligrams without a prescription.

At one time, P.A.B.A. was a chic substance, thought to prevent gray hair. That, plus its contraband status, gave it a certain amount of publicity, all very short-lived. Rinses and dyes, relatively inexpensive and needing no prescription, have proven considerably more effective.

C for Yourself

Vitamin C is one of the most popular of all the vitamins. Being water-soluble, it has to be taken every day, and its daily elimination in urine prevents the possibility of an overdose.

You can take a daily capsule or find plentiful supplies of vitamin C in citrus juices, particularly orange, grapefuit, and pineapple juices. One eight-ounce glass of orange juice provides about 130 milligrams of vitamin C; the recommended daily allowance is only forty-five milligrams daily. Though there is no known toxicity from taking too much vitamin C, over-consumption of any substance is courting trouble.

The most serious effect of a vitamin C deficiency is scurvy, which has been almost entirely eliminated from the western world. A mild deficiency often results in bleeding gums, easily bruised skin, wounds which require an inordinate time to heal, and chronic periods of fatigue often followed by muscle aches.

However, if one consumes at least the R.D.A. of vitamin C, one will be aiding the formation of red-blood cells and of collagen, an essential biological substance which helps to connect the cells of the body so they perform their proper function.

As yet there is no definitive evidence about vitamin C and its effect on the common cold, despite enthusiastic, partisan support for it.

Even more interesting than the sniffles are the experiments conducted on rats in a laboratory. One set of rats was deprived of vitamin C; the other was given adequate dosages. The rats deprived of vitamin C developed arteriosclerosis; the other group, receiving the R.D.A., had their blood cholesterol lowered.

D Truth and Nothing But D Truth

The most common source of vitamin D is milk that has been fortified with it, and a non-fat dry or skimmed milk is best. We do not recommend taking a supplement, unless it is medically prescribed, because a toxicity level exists.

If milk is not part of your diet, the sun provides a superb source of vitamin D. However, don't bathe immediately before or after exposure to the sun, for the oils of the skin's surface help to convert ultraviolet rays into vitamin D which is subsequently absorbed into the body. Without the presence of those natural oils, you will retain little or no vitamin D.

Vitamin D has been of inestimable value to the human race, greatly reducing, and in many areas completely eliminating, rickets. Vitamin D is also essential for the absorption and efficient utilization of calcium and phosphorus, which means strong bones and teeth.

The recommended daily allowance of vitamin D is 400 international units. More than that may be dangerous, in some cases even leading to death. Consumption of mounting quantities of vitamin D may initially result in a state of weakness and irritability; eventually, it deteriorates health with risky deposits of calcium in the blood.

E Gads

In the publicity stakes, vitamin E may be running neck and neck with vitamin C. Most health-conscious people are taking no chances; they're betting on both. While C has been touted as the answer to the common cold, E has received testimonials as an aphrodisiac as well as the best new heart medicine since the blood vessel.

Many laboratory experiments, on rats, have shown that vitamin E deficiencies have, indeed, resulted in sterility, miscarriages, anemia, and the degeneration of muscle tissues. Insufficient research has been conducted on humans, and a gaggle of nutritionists disagree on the precise value of vitamin E.

We do know that vitamin E plays an essential role in preventing oxygen from breaking down unsaturated fatty acids. The vitamin, itself, is also present in polyunsaturated fats, especially soybean oil, corn oil, and cottonseed oil. Unfortunately, it is easily and rapidly destroyed by cooking, freezing, and exposure to air. Small quantities can be found in unrefined grains, nuts, and wheat germ, especially when carefully stored.

The recommended daily allowance for adults is about fifteen international units.

The K Factor

Vitamin K has been justly regarded as vital for its sole function, to assist in the clotting of blood.

Because this vitamin is so common in just about every diet, deficiencies rarely exist. Excellent sources of vitamin K are raw cabbage, lettuce, leafy greens, broccoli, and spinach.

Mind Your Minerals

Minerals are essential to the healthy development and proper maturation of the body. As with vitamins, several minerals have recommended daily allowances, others do not. A wide range of nutritionists disagree on the actual R.D.A. of certain minerals, asserting that the quantities should be raised.

The majority of people do not require mineral supplements, unless so advised by a doctor. Most diets contain more than sufficient quantities of minerals. If you are taking a good multiple vitamin, you are probably getting additional minerals as well.

The Iron Works

The mineral iron is an essential element of hemoglobin, the oxygen-carrying agent in the red-blood cells. It is stored in various parts of the body, particularly in the marrow of the skeletal system, the liver, the spleen, and even in the muscles, where it is called myoglobin.

Iron is available from a wide variety of sources, including egg yolks, yeast, wheat germ, beef liver, leafy greens, whole grain, and most fish. The R.D.A. is ten milligrams per day for men and post-menopausal women. For most mature women, it is eighteen milligrams per day.

Because iron-deficiency anemia is common in women and adolescents, advertisers have concentrated their pitches at these two groups. Nevertheless, iron is essential to all diets, for both men and women. Since it is possible to take too much iron, check with a doctor before taking an iron supplement.

Have a Glass of Calcium

For generations, mothers have given their children milk, rich in calcium, so that they would have strong bones and teeth. And they have been right; calcium does, indeed, aid in the development of strong bones and teeth. But calcium is important even for the mature individual for it provides some insurance that bones and teeth will remain strong. Furthermore, it assists in the clotting of blood.

For an adequate supply of calcium, you must include vitamin D in your diet. Milk contains sufficient quantities of both. Unfortunately, many adults discontinue their milk intake, associating it with childhood. An eight-ounce glass of non-fat dry or skimmed milk will provide the calcium and vitamin D necessary for the strength and maintenance of adult bones and teeth and for effective self-repairs.

If you absolutely despise milk, try one container of yogurt every day.

During the week preceding menstruation, most women require more than the normal quantities of calcium; their calcium levels drop drastically. A calcium deficiency, during that week, will often result in depression and irritability. When menstruation begins, calcium levels drop even further, so that a woman should drink several glasses of milk each day.

Iodine at Home

The mineral iodine is essential to the proper functioning of the thyroid, an endocrine gland located in the neck, which affects the entire basal metabolism rate of the body. When the thyroid suffers a deficiency of iodine, the

170

basal metabolism rate slows down; when it speeds up, it is usually receiving excessive quantities of iodine.

Iodine helps in the formation of triiodothyronine and thyroxine, both vital hormones of the thyroid gland. If those hormones are not produced in adequate supply, there may be a quick weight gain, without even overeating. Other negative effects are fatigue, low blood pressure, and even goiter.

Fish, in general, provides adequate supplies of iodine, and iodized salt is one of the surest ways of getting iodine.

It Glows

Phosphorus works with calcium, converting various proteins into essential amino acids. The presence of vitamin D in the system is essential for both phosphorus and calcium to be properly and effectively absorbed.

Phosphorus, like calcium, helps to keep bones and teeth hard and also contributes to the proper functioning of muscles.

In the United States, as in most western countries, phosphorus deficiencies are rare because it is included in most well-balanced diets. The best sources of phosphorus are poultry, yogurt, non-fat dry and skimmed milk, and hard and soft cheese.

The Remainders

Other minerals are bromide, cholorine, chromium, copper, fluoride, magnesium, manganese, molybdenum, potassium, sodium, sulphur, and zinc. Well-balanced diets contain them all; deficiencies are rare.

Drink, Drank, and Drunk

More than ten million people in the United States recognize themselves as alcoholics; there are estimates of about ten million more with drinking problems who refuse to admit the truth either to themselves or to seek help.

Whether a social drinker or an alcoholic, it is important to know that alcohol destroys the nutritional value of many foods and is an arch villain of all the B vitamins. It impedes the proper funtioning of the liver, and eventually can destroy it completely, while reducing the optimum performance of the kidneys.

Alcohol affects people differently. Some people should have absolutely no alcohol and others can drink small amounts without suffering adverse effects. The many varieties of D.N.A. structures, which accounts for biological individuality, also accounts for the individual reaction.

Whatever your category, you need some general information about alcohol. For instance, vodka has no proteins, no carbohydrates, no fats, no vitamins, and no minerals. Still, a glass of 86 proof has 105 calories.

Wines contain small amounts of carbohydrates, calcium, vitamins B-1 and B-2, and a tiny quantity of niacin. Wine can range in calories from 85 to 140 per glass. Of all the alcoholic beverages, beer has the most nutrients, but no one would or should go on a diet of beer. A glass of beer contains 150 calories, as well as generous and fattening quantities of malt.

Alcohol can be fattening, yielding seven calories per gram, and it can injure your nutritional well-being, too. Alcohol often excites sexual desires, but it subsequently depresses sexual response. Alcoholism can and often does result in impotence as well as frigidity.

The point of all this frightening information is not to make everyone into a buttermilk addict, but to make people aware of the consequences of their own actions.

Weighed in the Balance

Most people are surprised to discover that one of us was once a fat gymnast. And it wasn't Jeffrey. Believe it or not, Suzy once weighed 160 pounds, and appeared on the September 1977 cover of *Weight Watchers* magazine. Through the Weight Watchers program, Suzy slimmed down to a stunning 112 pounds, going from a size fourteen to a size six, and has maintained that weight and size. It's not easy, but it can be done. It requires considerable effort, but it is an excellent investment in your body, your health, and most of all, in your self-esteem.

The Fat Figure

Obviously, we are believers in the Weight Watchers program; we regard it as far sounder than any of the fad diets. It is, quite simply, a plan for sensible eating, and one which has achieved remarkable results.

If you organize your own diet plan, we suggest you keep it simple. There is a basic principle to which you should adhere, based on a common-sense approach to dieting. Never consume more calories than you can burn up. Excess calories, if not burned up, have no place to go other than into layers of flab. If you lead a relatively sedentary life, you should be consuming far fewer calories than you did either as a child or as an active collegiate athlete. Even as active adults, we have found that our calorie intake is less than it was when we were teen-agers. We try to consume no more calories than we burn up, and we make sure we receive adequate quantities of vitamins and minerals. We try to eat well-balanced meals, highly nutritious and low in calories.

If you are careless about what you eat, you will suffer some form of malnutrition, and it may well be obesity, a continuous hazard to your very life. Excess weight is a peril to your heart, heartbeat, and blood pressure. Furthermore, it accelerates the aging process, while decreasing intellectual performance.

In his informative book, *Overweight Causes and Control*, Dr. Jean Mayer wrote, "Fat people are more likely to suffer from heart and kidney disease, high blood pressure, diabetes, and many other afflictions. Surgery is more hazardous when the patient is obese. . . . Excessive adipose tissue also adds to the problem of keeping the whole body oxygenated. Obese people have, accordingly, a diminished exercise tolerance and may show greater difficulty in normal breathing, particularly in the presence of any even mild respiratory infection. . . . Another condition where weight reduction is urgent is hypertension."

Obesity also has a negative affect on sexual responsiveness and skills. In men, excess fat may cause infertility if the folds of fatty tissue around the scrotum raise its temperature too high. Furthermore, it may lead to a less than absolutely rigid erection. In women, excess flab along the vaginal walls can reduce sensitivity. A related difficulty may be an irregular menstrual cycle. And in both sexes, a big belly may simply get in the way of completely satis-factory sexual intercourse.

Earlier we wrote that we try not to consume more calories than we burn up. And that is the most important principle for effective weight loss and weight maintenance.

If you work in an office, sitting behind a desk for seven or eight hours, you are leading a sedentary life and burning no more than 1,500 calories a day. A housewife will burn about the same number of calories. If you are a fireman, a football player, or an alligator wrestler, you will probably burn up about 3,500 calories a day. Yet most fairly inactive people consume 3,500 calories simply by eating and drinking between meals. They cannot avoid gaining weight, and that weight might be an extra twenty-five pounds.

Just imagine the burdens under which all of one's internal organs must operate. Heart, liver, and kidneys are all required to do more than is healthy for them. The body itself is carrying around all that extra weight, causing it to move slowly and lethargically.

If you are overweight, check our calorie chart to determine how many calories you burn daily. If you burn only 1,500 calories, you may choose to increase your activities, bringing your calorie expenditure up to 2,000. If that is the case, try to consume no more than 1,500 calories, until you have reached your optimum weight.

Don't begin any diet without a complete medical examination, followed by your doctor's suggestions for calorie intake and exercise.

Don't be too ambitious; weight should come off slowly and steadily. And sudden weight loss may have unfortunate, related results. If you can lose three pounds a week and keep them off, you have an excellent chance to maintain a good weight and good health.

Dieting is not a game of checkers with yourself; yet so many people play against themselves and cheat as well. If you are to be successful, you must be completely honest. Failure to admit the intake of extra calories will start you in a pattern of deception that will only add unwanted weight.

As the pounds come off, you don't want to be left with a flabby body. Therefore, our daily exercise program is an integral part of any diet plan. While dieting will limit calorie intake, exercise will firm and tone up your muscles, leaving you looking and feeling young and vigorous. And that is the purpose of this book. Good luck!

Calorie Utilization Chart

In any calorie utilization chart, cumulative figures are approximations only. It could not be otherwise, for each person has a different D.N.A. struc-ture, and each person exerts different amounts of effort to accomplish similar tasks. For instance, an unfit individual of sixty will probably burn up far 173 more calories while running for a bus than a teen-ager might while merely running for fun. In addition, calorie utilization is affected by weight, body type (ectomorph or endomorph), age, general fitness, and health.

So the activities listed on pages 175 and 176 reflect general amounts of calories, but they will serve the purpose of providing important guidelines. Calorie utilization is stated by activities and by hours as well. If you engage in the same activity every day for several months, the activity will become significantly easier, requiring a reduction of calories.

You will be able to judge your utilization and intake of calories by charting your weight daily, a procedure we strongly recommend.

CALORIE UTILIZATION CHART

Daily Activities	Per hour			Per week (1 hour a day)		
Eating	55	–	85	385	–	595
Dressing	25	–	100	175	–	700
Driving	100	–	150	700	–	1,050
Resting—supine	50	–	85	350	–	595
Sitting	25	–	50	175	–	350
Sleeping	30	–	70	210	–	490
Standing—at rest	20	–	80	140	–	560
Talking	75	–	100	525	–	700

Housework

	Per hour			Per week		
In general	200	–	300	1,400	–	2,100
Dusting	160	–	200	1,120	–	1,400
Making beds	200	–	250	1,400	–	1,750
Mopping	150	–	200	1,050	–	1,400
Polishing	200	–	250	1,400	–	1,750
Sewing	10	–	50	70	–	350
Sweeping	100	–	150	700	–	1,050
Washing dishes	60	–	100	420	–	700
Washing windows	225	–	275	1,575	–	1,925

Gardening

	Per hour			Per week		
In general	200	–	300	1,400	–	2,100
Hoeing & raking	250	–	325	1,750	–	2,275
Sawing wood	400	–	500	2,800	–	3,500
Shoveling snow	400	–	600	2,800	–	4,200
Weeding	250	–	325	1,750	–	2,275

Work

	Per hour			Per week		
Carpentry	150	–	300	1,050	–	2,100
Housepainting	150	–	225	1,050	–	1,575
Office work	150	–	225	1,050	–	1,575
Pick & shovel	300	–	600	2,100	–	4,200
Writing	25	–	100	175	–	700

Physical Exercise	Per hour	Per week (1 hour a day)
Walking 2 MPH	200 – 225	1,400 – 1,575
3 MPH	250 – 300	1,750 – 2,100
4 MPH	350 – 400	2,450 – 2,800
Jogging (under 5 MPH)	500 – 650	3,500 – 4,550
5.5 MPH	600 – 700	4,200 – 4,900
9 MPH	800 – 1,000	5,600 – 70,000
Cycling 5 MPH	250 – 300	1,750 – 2,100
10 MPH	450 – 500	3,150 – 3,500
15 MPH	650 – 800	4,550 – 5,600
Dancing	200 – 500	1,400 – 3,500
Sex	1,000 – 1,600	7,000 – 11,200

Sports

	Per hour	Per week (1 hour a day)
Calisthenics (medium)	250 – 400	1,750 – 2,800
(hard)	400 – 600	2,800 – 4,200
Baseball	300 – 500	2,100 – 3,500
Basketball	400 – 550	2,800 – 3,850
Bowling	200 – 400	1,400 – 2,800
Canoeing	175 – 500	1,225 – 3,500
Fencing	300 – 600	2,100 – 4,200
Golf	300 – 400	2,100 – 2,800
Handball (hard)	500 – 700	3,500 – 4,900
Horseback riding	150 – 600	1,050 – 4,200
Mountain climbing	600 – 900	4,200 – 6,300
Rowing (hard)	1,000 – 1,300	7,000 – 9,100
Sailing	150 – 600	1,050 – 4,200
Skating	300 – 600	2,100 – 4,200
Skiing	250 – 550	1,750 – 3,850
Soccer	525 – 600	3,675 – 4,200
Squash	600 – 800	4,200 – 5,600
Swimming (breaststroke)	300 – 600	2,100 – 4,200
(crawl)	500 – 700	3,500 – 4,900
Tennis (doubles)	400 – 500	2,800 – 3,500
(singles)	550 – 700	3,850 – 4,900
Volleyball	300 – 600	2,100 – 4,200

Weight Chart

Look at the sample weight chart on this page and mark yours accordingly. Try to weigh yourself at the same time every morning; before breakfast is the best time. If you don't want to weigh yourself every day, weight yourself once a week, but do it on the same day of the week. Consistency is absolutely essential to the success of any program.

WEIGHT CHART

Date
started

Weight
date
started

Mark in your weight on starting day. Then mark in five pounds going up the chart and nine pounds going down. Keep track of your weight loss or gain.

Example chart shows a steady black line and two broken lines. The steady line is an example of a good weight loss. The two broken lines are examples of erratic eating habits and therefore are not good.

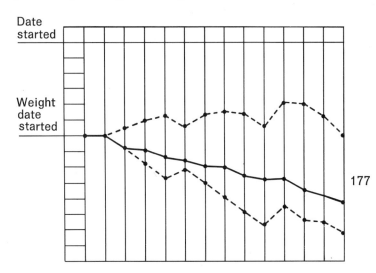

Date
started

Weight
date
started

177

Count Your Calories Chart

The total number of calories you eat each day may surprise you. From the chart on page 179, you will learn what foods to keep in your diet and which ones to eliminate.

Follow the example at the top of the chart and write in everything you eat each day. Even if it's only a taste of something, you must enter it; small tastes add up to a significant amount of calories. Write in the number of calories; then total up your caloric intake at the end of the day. If you are gaining weight, cut out some of the food; if you are maintaining your optimum weight, then you are consuming the right number of calories for your body. If you are losing weight, then you are consuming fewer calories than your body is burning up. Most important, be sure you eat a well-balanced diet, one which will not overload your system leaving you with either superfluous calories or insufficient nutrition.

CALORIE COUNTER—FOOD INTAKE CHART

	Breakfast	Snack	Lunch	Snack	Dinner	Snack	Total
Example	coffee 2 eggs (boiled) ½ grapefruit	vanilla yogurt 3 oz.	veg. soup tuna salad 3 oz. mayo.	apple	4 oz. chick. asparagus salad, dr.	fruit salad bite of Jeffrey's choc. mousse (50)	
	150 75	180	82 250	80	300 150 150 150	350	1917
Monday							
Tuesday							
Wednesday							
Thursday							
Friday							
Saturday							
Sunday							

Keep track of everything you put in your mouth. For better results, carry a small notebook wherever you go and mark in it whatever you eat.

Index